Powers of Healing

Powers of Healing

By the Editors of Time-Life Books

TIME-LIFE BOOKS, ALEXANDRIA, VIRGINIA

CONTENTS

CHAPTER 1

Other Roads to Health

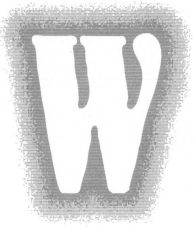

hen noted writer and editor Norman Cousins returned home from a trip abroad in the summer of 1964, he had a slight fever and a general feeling of malaise. Soon achiness and a deadening fatigue settled in his joints, and within a week he was having difficulty moving. Cousins consulted his physician and, after exhaustive tests, was diagnosed as having ankylosing spondylitis, a devastating form of arthritis that attacks the body's connective tissue. Victims of the malady are plagued by a progressive, immobilizing welding of the joints of the spine, ribs, neck, and jaw. Cousins's case was especially severe, and he was given only a 1 in 500 chance of survival. Despite this almost certain death sentence, he determined to wage a heroic struggle against the disease.

In the 1979 bestseller *Anatomy of an Illness As Perceived by the Patient,* a personal narrative of his experience, Norman Cousins professed a lifelong interest in medical science. He had read widely in the history of medicine and had been intrigued by studies on the effects of placebos—those dummy drugs that have no intrinsic value but nevertheless can sometimes work through the power of suggestion, healing patients who trust in them. Cousins also subscribed to the belief that emotions play an active role in one's state of health. He was particularly intrigued by organic chemist Hans Selye's classic 1956 work, *The Stress of Life,* which examined the damage that stress and negative emotions can do to body chemistry. "The inevitable question arose in my mind," Cousins wrote. "What about the positive emotions? If negative emotions produce negative chemical changes in the body, wouldn't positive emotions produce positive chemical changes? Is it possible that love, hope, faith, laughter, confidence, and the will to live have positive therapeutic value?"

Cousins decided to systematically pursue the positive as an antidote to the worst psychological symptoms of his illness—panic and helplessness. In partnership with his physician, who continued to administer basic medical care, Cousins developed what he called "an auspicious environment . . . for recovery." One of its more interesting components was "laugh therapy"— daily doses of Marx Brothers' films, humor books, and the like—which not only helped ease his pain and allow him peaceful sleep, but also seemed to improve his blood chemistry. In addition, Cousins persuaded his doctor to let him leave the hospital and move into a hotel, where he could rest undisturbed. Eight days after Cousins had assumed an active role in his own care, his astonished doctor could measure genuine progress against the disease. And although a near-total recovery took years to complete, Cousins was able to return to work full time only four months after beginning his unorthodox regimen.

Skeptics claim that Norman Cousins's remarkable tale of recovery raises serious questions about the accuracy of his doctor's initial diagnosis. But Cousins and many others think it vividly demonstrates the mysterious ways in which the interactions of mind and body—and some say spirit—may affect health. While the mind-body connection is recognized by Western medicine as one factor in the health equation, it constitutes the basic tenet of many healing techniques practiced outside of the medical mainstream. Often grouped under the broad heading "alternative therapies," these methods range from time-honored techniques such as acupuncture, homeopathy, and the laying on of hands to such newfangled New Age treatments as crystal and aroma therapies.

Advocates of Western medicine place these treatments outside medicine's scientific arena and in a realm all their own, one that is, for the most part, impervious to government regulation and therefore potentially dangerous. But practitioners of alternative therapies argue that they are simply harking back to an earlier time, trying to recapture the wisdom of the ancients, pursuing healing methods more natural than the "magic bullets" prescribed by Western physicians. Proponents of alternative therapies claim a philosophical rapport with healers from many cultures, past and present. Although the curative techniques may range from the ecstatic spirit dances of shamans to the somnolent

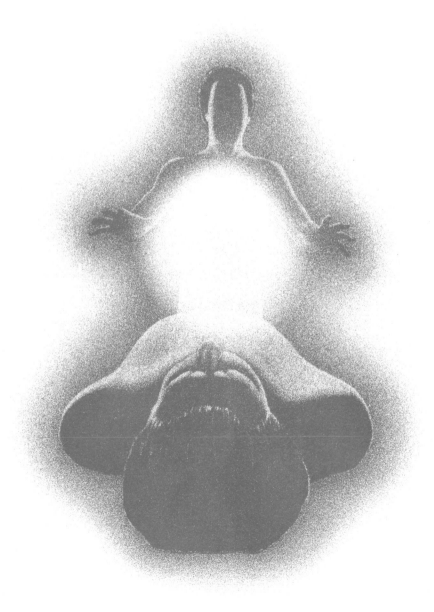

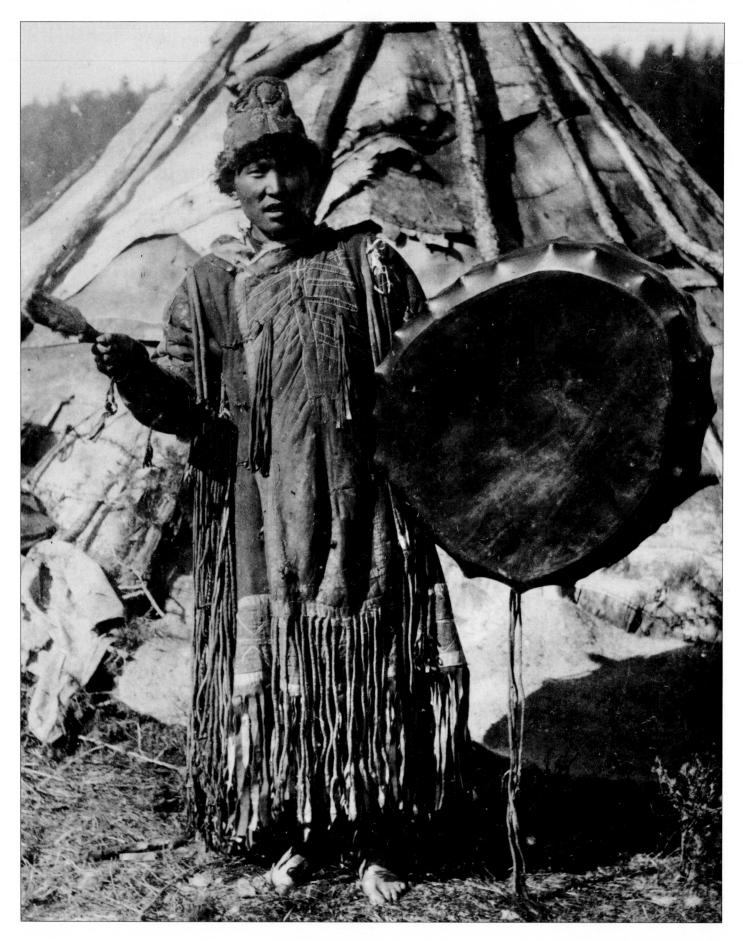

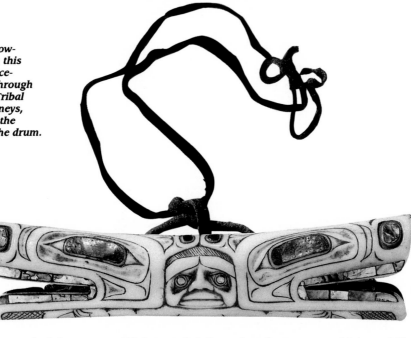

Tulayev, shaman of Siberia's now-extinct Karagass tribe, poses in this 1927 photograph with his trance-inducing reindeer-skin drum, through which spirits allegedly spoke. Tribal lore held that on its astral journeys, Tulayev's soul rode the soul of the reindeer whose skin provided the drum.

trances of "Sleeping Prophet" Edgar Cayce, from the practices of faith healers to those of shiatsu massage therapists, most of the practitioners share an underlying belief that mind, body, and spirit are inextricably connected. Health, according to their system of thinking, is a state of harmony or balance among the forces—energies, gods, or spirits—thought to govern the whole being. Sickness is a contrary state of disease or conflict among those forces. The idea is hardly unique to this century; it recalls millenniums-old Chinese and Indian traditions that imply the same conclusion: All ailments, from the common cold to cancer, are symptoms of more profound disruptions in the inner being. The goal of alternative healers, then, is to relieve the suffering individual by restoring harmony, the normal state of existence, and with it, health.

This bone and shell "soul catcher" was used by North America's Tlingit Indians, who believed illness resulted from the soul's being magically lured from the body. Tlingit shamans used the device to suck up air from around the sick person and blow the captured soul back into the body.

Scientific medicine, which began to gain ground in the eighteenth century and became the dominant mode of healing in the industrial West in the mid-nineteenth century, has traditionally taken a dim view of such alternative approaches to healing. Generations of physicians who were trained to be skilled mechanics of the human body, who understood disease to be a breakdown in the operation of a finely tuned engine, could find no rational explanation for cures achieved through other means. They were understandably troubled that unorthodox methods were seldom measured, quantified, or examined empirically. Thus physicians and scientists felt compelled to deny the claims of those subscribing to alternative healing and to denigrate the practitioners, even though many of the naysayers knew from their own experience that patients and diseases did not always behave in the exact way textbooks said they should.

Early in the twentieth century, though, discoveries first in psychology and then in neurology, biochemistry, and immunology, all of which *could* be tested scientifically, began to cast fresh light on the nature of sickness and health. New research showed that chronic emotional problems can sometimes find outlets in physical ailments, that specific diseases such as rheumatoid arthritis and high blood pressure can be triggered by stress, that heart rate and pulse can be manipulated through conscious effort using a process called biofeedback, that certain treatments such as massage and acupuncture can sometimes elicit specific therapeutic responses, that pain can be controlled not only by attitude—an astounding fact in itself—but by chemicals called endorphins that are released in moments of high stress or excitement, that placebos can be as effective as the medicines they imitate; and the list goes on.

These surgical tools were used by a shaman of the Chukchi peoples of northeastern Siberia. The iron knife (right) sports a glass bead, supposedly a gift from the spirits. Leather effigies of evil spirits subdued by the shaman dangle from the oblong ivory knife.

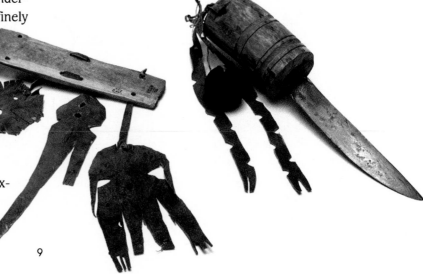

It seemed that some kind of reconciliation between healers and physicians was due. Yet despite their increasing recognition of the mind-body-spirit health connection and the efforts by many physicians to consider all three in their treatments, the medical establishment remained skeptical. Scientists cite several rationales to explain away alternative therapies' apparent successes. Many diseases are self-limiting, they say, and with or without intervention by doctor or healer, they will be cured by the body's own defenses. Other illnesses may enter periods of spontaneous remission, lying dormant for a time, confounding those who predict their statistical courses. And then there are the psychosomatic sicknesses, originating in the mind but manifesting themselves in the body—which can disappear with only a change in thought or attitude.

Thus the line is drawn between Western medicine and alternative therapies. Medicine demands scientific proof of the alternative systems, while the acupuncturists and herbalists and trance healers point to their apparent successes as proof enough.

If we are to believe the indirect evidence of cave paintings and odd bits of artifacts in places as far apart as southern Africa and eastern Siberia, the roots of trance healing—the oldest of therapies—go back perhaps 40,000 years to the healer-priests who served the scattered tribes of Stone Age hunter-gatherers. Known as shamans, a term that originated with North Asian, Ural-Altaic, and Paleo-Asian peoples but is now broadly used, such healers still exist as a religious and cultural phenomenon among many tribal societies. They enjoy a position of respect in a variety of native cultures in the Americas, central Asia, Africa, southeast India, and Australia. And it is from studying these latter-day examples that ethnologists have formed a fairly detailed picture of the shaman's function.

The shaman is essentially a practitioner of white, or good, magic, who uses his or her gifts to mediate between the spirit forces of an often hostile cosmos and the people. In many tribes, the shaman is regarded as semidivine, resid-

ing in the material world but able to travel at will to other worlds to communicate freely with spirits. These special qualities oblige the shaman to know matters relevant to humankind's survival but hidden from ordinary mortals. (The word *shaman* is derived from the Tunguso-Manchurian word *saman,* "to know.") In many ways, this healer is the ultimate psychic, for many shamans claim the power to see distant time and place (clairvoyance and precognition), to read human thought (telepathy), and to intercede in all matters of physical and mental health (psychic healing).

Like every other aspect of existence in the shamanistic societies, illness is seen as a phenomenon beyond human control. It is thought to originate in a wide variety of causes, ranging from the malevolence of an angry god, the breaking of a taboo, or the power of a magic spell to spirit possession, the loss of one's soul, or the imbalance of some elemental forces. The first test of any shaman, then, is whether he or she can discover the supernatural reason for the sickness. Some sicknesses have traditionally identifiable signs and symptoms and conventional shamanistic cures. But often, the disease that overtakes the shaman's patient is believed to be disguised, and in order to treat it, the healer must travel to the spirit world for guidance.

Shamans claim to communicate with the spirits through some form of mind alteration. Every shamanistic culture has its own prescribed rituals for achieving this state, but they are all likely to include sleep deprivation, sexual abstinence, and fasts, followed by dancing, the repetitious chanting of magical words and phrases, the prolonged and hypnotic beating of drums, and at times the taking of hallucinogenic substances—the amanita mushroom by some Siberian shamans, for example, and peyote by the Huichol Indian shamans of Mexico. Certain shamans fall into what psychologists call the passive state of ecstasy, in which the body struggles desperately against the spirits, only to succumb as possession overtakes it; thereafter, the unconscious shaman becomes the mouthpiece for the spirit. Other shamans adopt the role of "wandering ecstatic":

The body functions slow to a minimum, and the shaman appears to die; his soul is then said to journey to the spirits for knowledge and to return as the shaman awakes to tell what has been learned.

Most shamanistic rituals are carried out at night, by firelight, in a place designated as sacred—in a cave, by a spring, or on a mountaintop. The sick person is part of the performance, but so too are the rest of the clan or village, who frequently join in the ceremonial singing, dancing, and chanting. The shaman wears symbolic garb and carries a deep-throated drum, a drumstick, perhaps a rattle, and a shaman mirror. The whole performance may last from sev-eral hours to several days, as the fantastic figure moves with gathering force through the healing ritual.

Psychologists who have studied shamanism in depth regard the entire process as therapeutic. The fact that the shaman agrees to treat the patient creates in the sufferer the expectation of recovery, for shamans are said to choose intuitively those diseases that are most likely to respond to their brand of medicine. Add to this the shaman's general reputation for omniscience, the spectators' collective confidence and good will, and the patient's belief that he or she is no longer battling evil spirits alone, and most of the ingredients exist for reducing the emotional stress that is now known to play a part in so many illnesses. However, the shaman's healing magic does not stop there. Clients are often given one or more specialized therapies, the healing values of which have also been scientifically confirmed in recent years. These include forms of relaxation and massage, herbs and dietary prescriptions, visualization, exorcism, ritual cleansing, confession, hypnosis, and the use of placebos.

Shamans do not usually choose their vocation but are called to it in a powerful way—through an extraordinarily vivid dream of possession, a vision quest (the deliberate seeking of direction from a spirit), or the trials of severe illness and recovery. The shaman's rite of passage, which is sometimes a public ceremony but may just as likely be a personal conversion, concludes with an experience of symbolic death and resurrection: The shaman-elect may ascend the "world tree" and pass into the celestial realm, thereby shedding his earthbound status. Then the neophyte receives instruction from a master shaman or from

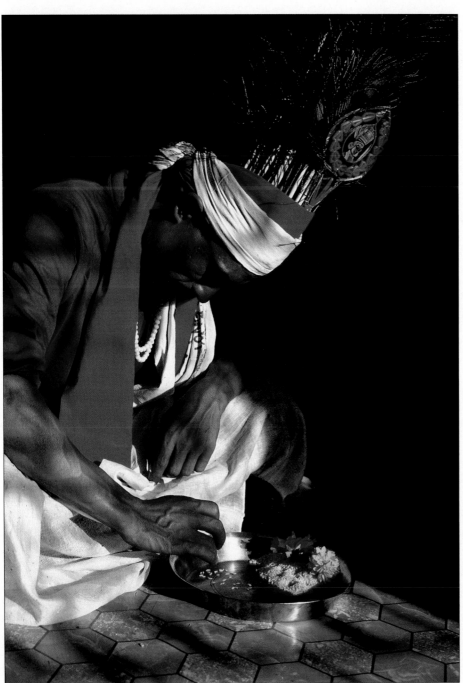

A Nepalese shaman matches grains of rice on a brass plate while chanting mantras, all part of an ancient diagnostic rite that seeks to divine the cause of a patient's disease. If the ritual fails, the shaman will enter a trance, become possessed, and consult directly with the spirit world about the illness's origins.

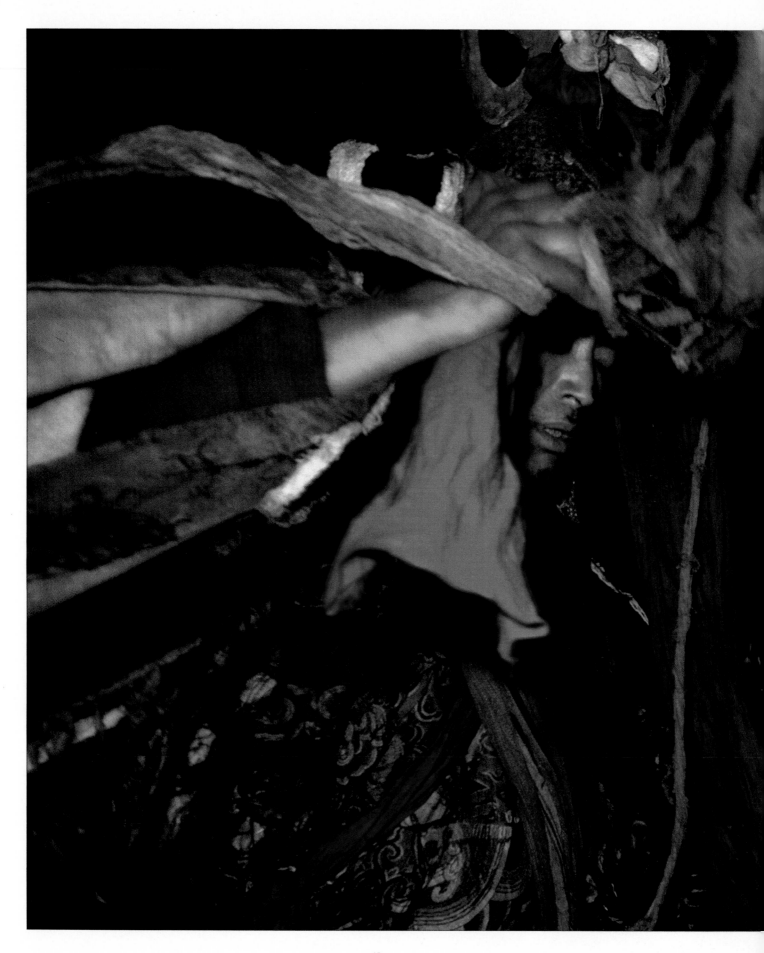

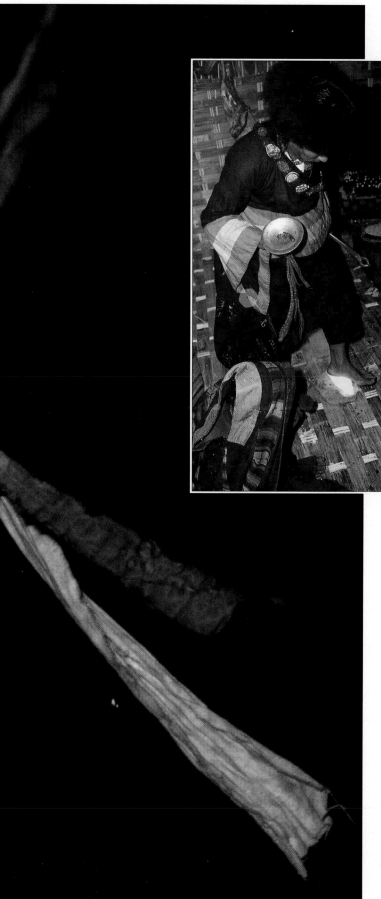

In the Tsangbu Valley between Nepal and Tibet, a shaman dances in metaphorical combat with a demon. Streamers flying from the shaman's headdress are said to help him contact gods and spirits. Dance is used to induce shamanistic trances in many cultures; often the shaman then proves the trance is complete. For example, another Tsangbu shaman (inset) stamps barefoot on a piece of white-hot metal. His imperviousness to pain confirms his trance state.

the spirits in the craft of healing, including the use of medicinal herbs and the prayers, songs, and chants that are the fundamental elements of the ceremonies.

For thousands of years, through the ancient civilizations of Sumer and Egypt, of Ur and Babylonia, priests conceived in the shaman mold continued to be the agents of public healing among increasingly sophisticated societies—a tribute, perhaps, to how good their brand of psychology mixed with simple therapeutics was. These latter-day shamans worked their healing magic as they always had, according to divine inspiration, although as time went on their rituals and diagnoses tended to become more specialized. Ancient papyri reveal, for example, that the incantations and medications of ancient Egypt varied from disease to disease and that cures often called for the patient's wearing of some kind of amulet, which might be a clay or wooden image, a string of beads, a knotted cord, or a stone.

Even the ancient Greeks had their shamanistic equivalents. Chief among their healing gods was Aesculapius, the offspring of Apollo. Using knowledge of the healing arts as taught him by his father and the wise centaur Chiron, Aesculapius had served mankind as a human shaman. But the god's extraordinary gifts proved his undoing. When he had all but abolished sickness and death, Pluto, god of the Underworld, complained that "the supply of new souls to the Shades is being endangered by all this healing." Zeus promptly had Aesculapius struck with a thunderbolt.

Many temples were erected to the slain healer's memory, and the sick flocked to these sacred places, called *asklepieia,* seeking relief. The individual would make a sacrificial offering, take a purifying bath, and participate in a solemn service of prayer. One or more priests would then question the sufferer closely about any dreams that had occurred before the symptoms or in the days since, in search of clues to

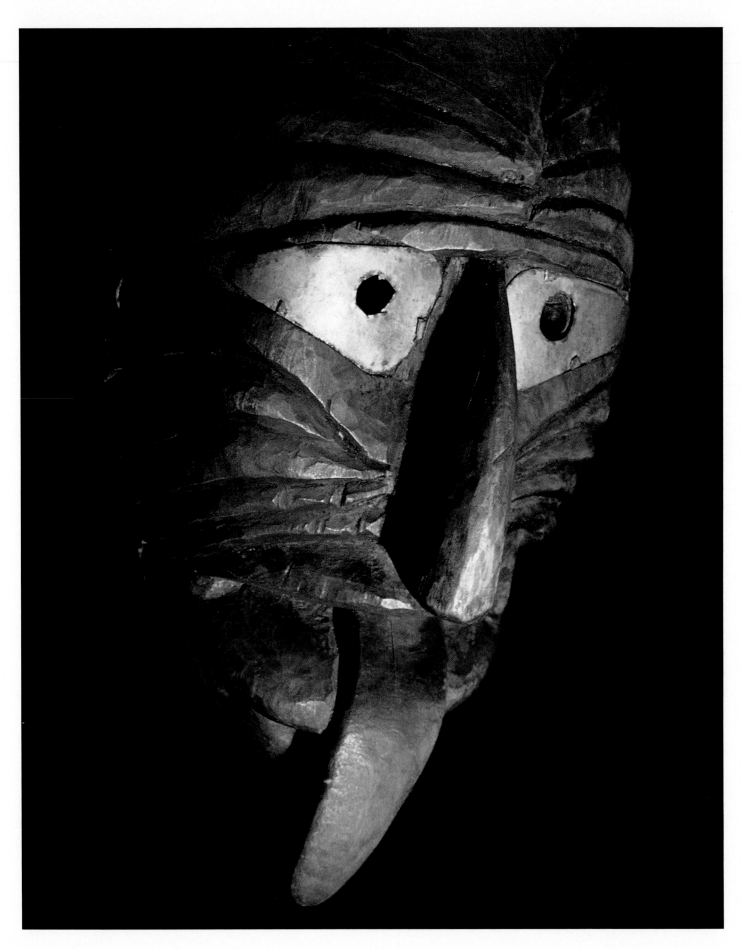

the nature of the illness. The individual would bed down for the night on the *abaton,* the colonnaded terrace surrounding the temple, to await a visit from Aesculapius, who might either speak in a dream or cure the petitioner outright. In time, the person would be awakened by one of the priests and, after further rituals and incantations, sent on his or her way.

Inscriptions engraved on the stone tablets at the asklepieia at Epidaurus suggest that many of the sick experienced dramatic improvements. One legend tells of the warrior Enippos who "had for six years the point of a spear in his cheek. As he was sleeping the god extracted the spearhead and gave it to him into his hands." Another reports that "Hermodites of Lamosakos was paralysed in body. In his sleep he was healed by the god, who ordered him to bring to the temple as large a stone as he could when he left the abaton. The man brought the stone, which now lies before the abaton."

The cult of Aesculapius flourished unchallenged until the end of the fifth century BC, when that extraordinary figure known as the Father of Medicine, Hippocrates of Cos, appeared on the scene. Contrary to the established doctrine of the era, Hippocrates was convinced that illness was a natural process, quite devoid of magic, and that a skillful physician using only his powers of observation could differentiate one disease from another. Like other Greek philosophers, Hippocrates believed that human beings were an orderly part of an orderly cosmos and that just as there were four phases of the moon, four cardinal points of the earth, four winds in the heavens, and four elements on earth, there were correspondences in the body—four "humors" (blood; phlegm; yellow choler; and melancholy, or black choler) and four "qualities" (dryness, dampness, heat, and cold). Health depended on the proper balance of humors and qualities; sickness was the natural consequence of an imbalance.

Hippocrates thought a doctor's chief service to the patient was in providing the prerequisite conditions through which the healing power of nature might work most effectively. Those conditions consisted primarily of a regimen of rest, attentive nursing, proper diet, exercise, and fresh air. From time to time, Hippocrates also recommended the sparing use of drugs—he recognized over 300 healing plants—as well as enemas, purges, diuretics, or bleeding, if the body seemed unable to bring about its own cure. But even with his more rational approach, Hippocrates always maintained a modest opinion of how much the physician could know or do alone. "Life is short, art is long, opportunity fleeting, experiment deceptive, and judgment difficult," he is believed to have written, adding that in order to effect a cure "the patient, and everyone else who is involved in the situation, must cooperate."

Hippocrates and his followers redirected the thrust of Western healing, turning it away from the spiritual and toward the physical causes of disease. For centuries, urban, if not rural, medicine in the

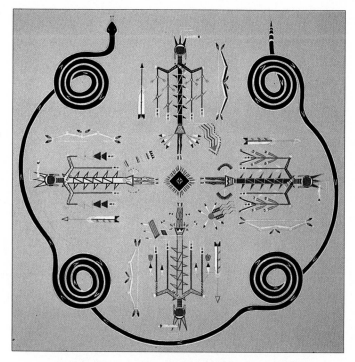

The Navajo believed that depicting gods in sand paintings could enlist their aid in restoring good health. This 1936 watercolor is a reproduction of a sand picture that is called **Endless Snake and Wind People.** *Navajos slept atop such sacred art in order to cure insomnia, tension, and other ills.*

Greek world and later in the Roman Empire developed along quasi-scientific lines. The second-century Greek physician Galen, an intellectual descendant of Hippocrates, did much to advance pharmacological knowledge in particular. But with the establishment of Christianity as the official religion of Rome in the fourth century, knowledge of "secular" medicine was shelved, literally, in the great library at Alexandria and underwent no significant improvement in the West for a thousand years.

In medieval Europe, the Christian clergy held a virtual monopoly on the practice of healing, and stories of miraculous cures were among the principal enticements that Christian missionaries would use in order to draw converts to the faith. And the philosophical basis for healing was not unlike that of shamanistic societies: Sickness and disease were the work of demons that took possession of the body—except that now the demons were agents of the devil rather than animist spirits.

Clergymen, who were God's agents on earth and whose life of contemplation was said to give them special knowledge of his healing powers, were the logical persons to consult when sickness overwhelmed the body or mind. Every man or woman of the cloth could, in theory, mediate healing. But those possessed of charisma, who had experienced visions, who knew states of ecstasy, or who claimed

Folk healing invades a technological sanctum as Papago medicine man Sam Angelo uses his shaman's rattle to minister to a fellow tribesman in a reservation hospital in Sells, Arizona. Staff doctors cooperate with Angelo, respecting his traditional tribal methods.

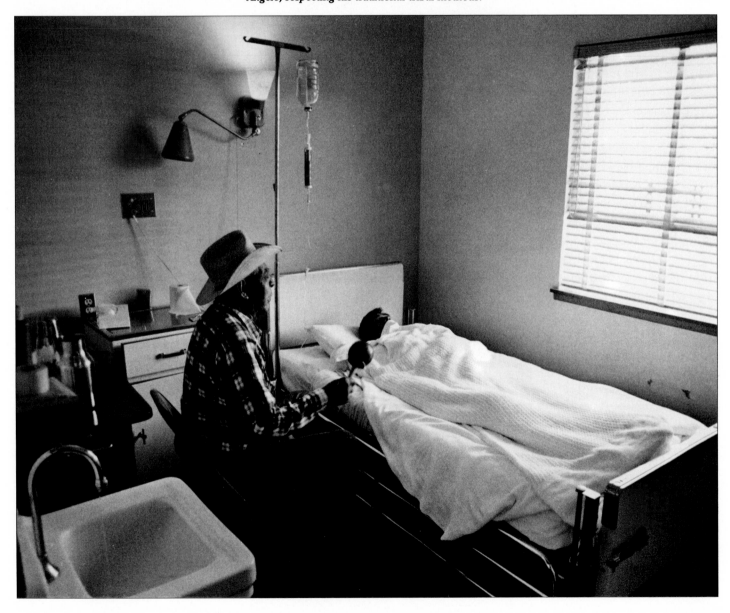

mystic intuition were clear favorites in that they were by definition closer to the Almighty. Like the shamans, these charismatics inspired in their clients the kind of trust and autosuggestion essential to effective spiritual healing. Treatment consisted of prayers, ritual gestures and chants, exorcism, the laying on of hands, and the touching of holy relics, all activities for which there was ample precedent in the lives of Jesus and the Apostles.

All things considered, the record of these early Christian healers seems to have been a positive one. Church documents indicate that thousands of cure seekers experienced improvements, even full cures, and in the process became living testimonials to the powers of faith and to the particular expertise of the healer who had delivered them from Satan. The unfortunate minority who did not get better were presumed to be stubborn, persistently sinful, lacking in faith, or otherwise irredeemable in God's eyes.

Although most of the medieval healers remain anonymous, one whose name and works endured is the German mystic Hildegard of Bingen. Born in 1098, the tenth child of a family of the minor nobility, Hildegard appeared from an early age to be one endowed with great gifts. At three years old, she claimed to have been visited by a dazzling white light. Although she was too young to even describe it at the time, Hildegard would soon recognize that light as the hallmark of the visions that would come to her regularly throughout her life. And through those visions, Hildegard was said to be able to foretell the future—at the tender age of five years, she astonished her nurse by looking at a pregnant cow and accurately predicting the markings of the unborn calf.

Perhaps because of her peculiar waking dreams, Hildegard's parents tithed her to God at the age of eight. (During the Middle Ages, it was common for the nobility to offer into monasticism children who were deemed unable to lead "normal" lives because of some handicap.) The young girl went to live at a tiny Benedictine convent, Saint Disibod, near Kreuznach in the Rhine Valley. She settled happily into life there, confiding her mysterious visions only to her mistress and surrogate parent, Jutta of Sponheim.

After Jutta's death in 1136, Hildegard, an extremely pious young woman, succeeded to the leadership of her convent. Five years later, at the age of forty-two, she reportedly received her calling as a prophet—again, through a vision. For the first time, she began recording the countless images that would inform the rest of her life.

Describing her unique trancelike experiences to another cleric years afterward, Hildegard wrote, "I have always seen this vision in my soul. . . . I do not hear them with my outward ears, nor do I perceive them by the thoughts of my own heart or by any combination of my five senses, but in my soul alone, while my outward eyes are open. So I have never fallen prey to ecstacy in the visions, but I see them wide awake, day and night. The light I see thus is not spacial, but it is far brighter than a cloud that carries the sun. I can measure neither height, nor length, nor breadth in it; and I call it 'the reflection of the living Light.' And as the sun, the moon, and the stars appear in water, so writings, sermons, virtues, and certain human actions take form for me and gleam within it."

Today, researchers convincingly argue that what passed for Hildegard's visions were, in fact, the auras of migraine headaches. Nonetheless, many contemporary healers and followers of today's so-called New Age have embraced Hildegard enthusiastically, exalting her as a prophet and a healer. During her life, Hildegard wrote a number of medically oriented books, including *Causae et Curae,* a treatise on clinical medicine. She never specifically credited her visions for the content of those works, as she would for other books, but simply maintained that all her knowledge of healing was through God's words. "In all creation, trees, plants, animals, and gem stones, there are hidden secret powers which no person can know of unless they are revealed by God," she declared. Health she knew to be just another manifestation of the individual's oneness with God, who is the source of all life and vitality. Disease was, conversely, the work of Satan, the embodiment of all evil. It

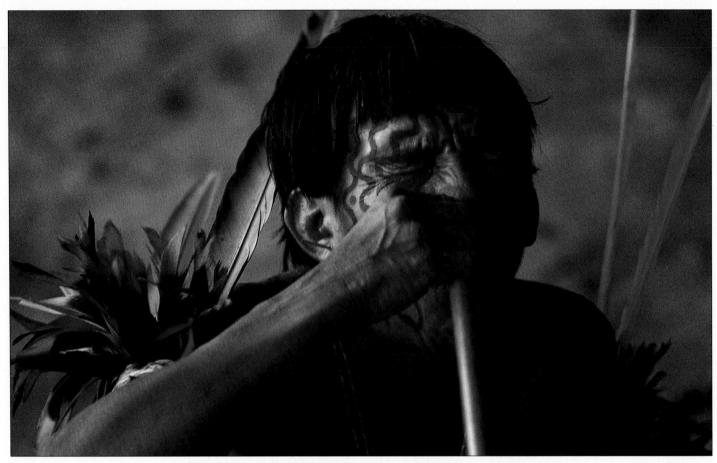

In the primal fastness of the Amazon rain forest, a Yanomami Indian shaman sniffs a powerful hallucinogen made from powdered tree bark. Under the drug's influence, he will seek spirit help to diagnose and cure the sick.

was Satan, she believed, who separated men from God, and in this separateness humankind becomes exposed to cosmic and atmospheric influences that can disrupt the perfect harmony that once existed among "the basic building blocks of the cosmos" in each of us—fire, air, water, and earth. By Hildegard's reckoning, there were twenty-four ways in which the fluids of the four world elements could become disharmonious, and these various combinations showed themselves in twenty-four basic illnesses. The healing force that could set them to rights she termed *viriditas,* literally "greenness" but symbolically the principle of life energy and creation.

Hildegard's treatments were not the sort to produce overnight cures or back-from-the-grave miracles. Rather, they were largely prescriptions for living a good life, spiritually and physically, so that a person could once again regain cosmic harmony. The majority of the abbess's remedies called for a combination of dietary moderation, spiritual reaffirmation, and perhaps a dose of high-fiber whole grain. Hildegard also regarded various precious stones as useful in treatment, a theory embraced by many of today's New Age

healers. As she explained it, the archangel Lucifer had once adorned himself magnificently with fiery stones. But when he joined forces with Satan and was cast out of Heaven, the gems fell from his garments and scattered over the earth where they remain as "an honor and blessing." Thereafter, whenever Satan/Lucifer caught sight of such stones, it was such a painful reminder of his lost magnificence that he immediately fled, making them efficacious in managing certain diseases.

Hildegard recommended that persons suffering from glaucoma or other painful eye problems should hold a piece of lapis lazuli in the mouth before breakfast, moisten it with saliva, then rub the saliva on the eyes to get relief. Lapis lazuli, dipped in wine three times, was also good to quench a rejected suitor's "blazing lust." Jasper, warmed with breath, could be put into the outer ear to restore hearing; water or wine in which a diamond had been soaked banished jaundice, and chalcedony was good for a troublesome gall bladder and for the anger produced by black bile.

In addition to her books on health, the abbess authored several others that she claimed were written in col-

Salvaging from the Jungle Sages

Ethnobotany is a new science whose mission is to rescue an old one—to salvage the herbal medical lore of jungle shamans before encroaching civilization destroys both their preserves and their knowledge.

Among the earliest ethnobotanists was venturesome Nicole Maxwell *(below),* who literally stumbled into the field. The daughter of a privileged San Francisco family, Maxwell dabbled in medicine and several other studies, was married and divorced, and at age forty was still restlessly searching for her true calling when she set out to explore the wilds of South America. One day in 1952, she tripped and fell on her machete in a Peruvian jungle, cutting her arm. A tourniquet failed to staunch the blood flow, so she accepted an Indian remedy—some dark liquid that was both taken orally and applied to the wound. The bleeding, she reported later, stopped in about three minutes.

For the next four decades, Maxwell made many more jungle forays to collect flora used in South American Indian folk medicine. She recorded her adventures in

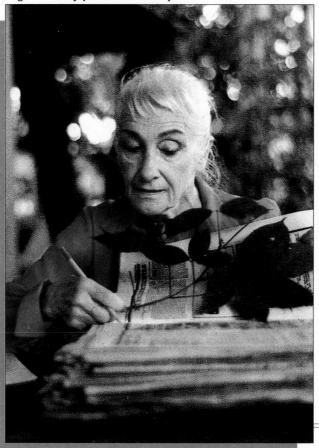

a 1961 book, *Witch Doctor's Apprentice.*

What she lacked in academic credentials, Maxwell made up in curiosity, enthusiasm, and faith in her work. Of the hundreds of plants she amassed, she reckoned that at least thirty could provide treatments that currently lie beyond modern medicine. She found, for instance, that a sedge called the *piripiri* was used by several tribes as a highly effective oral contraceptive. Given to a girl at puberty, the drug apparently prevented conception for six to

seven years. There were also plant concoctions that seemed able to promote fertility, stop internal bleeding, prevent tooth decay, allow the extraction of teeth without pain or bleeding, dissolve kidney stones, and cause fast and scarless healing of burns.

One drug company backed a Maxwell expedition and promised to research her findings. It finally became clear, however, that the company's real interest was in the promotional value of a stylish woman hacking through jungles for native cures. No effort was made to test or exploit her discoveries.

But attitudes are changing. Since ethnobotany began in the 1930s and 1940s, herbal healing has yielded proven tools, among them digitalis for heart failure, curare as a muscle relaxant, and vincristine for treating leukemia. And more dedicated scientists are entering the field, even as the earth's tropical rain forests are being decimated. Their hope is that the unwritten wisdom of the shamans, passed down orally through long generations, can be saved before the witch doctors vanish along with the jungles.

laboration with God. These included *Scivias,* which prophesied "a regenerated world [in which] the angels will return with confidence to dwell among men." Hildegard's works brought her to the attention of no less a personage than Pope Eugene III, who praised her at the Trier synod of 1147. Thereafter, her fame spread throughout the Continent, and pilgrims flocked to the tiny Benedictine monastery to which her convent was connected. She soon persuaded patrons to build her a new and larger cloister in Rupertsberg, near the city of Bingen, and there, for the duration of her long and apparently luminous life, she received those seeking cures and spiritual counseling. Hildegard died on September 17, 1179, and it was said that on that night the heavens received her gladly, the stars arraying themselves in the form of a cross.

Faith healing continued, gradually diminishing, in the centuries following Hildegard's death. Its decline followed many social changes, including that intractable human health disaster known as the Black Death and the rise of secular humanism, a philosophy exalting man's life and potential on earth, rather than the expectations for his soul after death. As the Renaissance gained momentum, classical medicine was revived and the medical arts were reestablished on a scientific footing. The great work on human anatomy by Flemish biologist Andreas Vesalius appeared in 1543; more reliable translations of ancient medical texts—particularly those by Hippocrates and Galen—became available; and exploration of new lands brought new drugs into use. Alternative healing, to the extent that it was practiced, became the province of kings and princes, who were said to have the royal touch—the ability to cure disease by merely touching the afflicted. In this unsympathetic climate, other unconventional "cures" were far more likely to come from cynical quacks, charlatans, and pseudoscientists than from faith healers.

Little changed until the early years of the nineteenth century, when a new liberalism swept over every aspect of society, from religious beliefs to scientific dogma. Nowhere was this optimism more pervasive or more productive of mystic cults and faiths than in the United States. In the young nation's heady social and philosophical atmosphere, some thinkers began to wonder if the mind, properly trained to its transcendental possibilities, might not actually be capable of perceiving a reality beyond all physical phenomena. The Spiritualist movement that swept from New England's shores to the farthest frontiers of the West beginning in the 1840s was based on this premise. And one of the first to herald its arrival was a young trance healer named Andrew Jackson Davis.

Davis, who came to be known as the Poughkeepsie Seer, was born in 1826 in the small town of Blooming Grove, New York. His mother was an uneducated, careworn woman who found her refuge in religion, and his father was a sometime weaver, cobbler, and farm laborer who spent most of his sporadic earnings on rum. Davis would later describe his dreary home life as one of "ignorance, intemperance, poverty and discord." About the only encouraging words he heard as a child issued from a mysterious, disembodied voice that spoke in tones "very low, clear, sweet, dreamy, influential." The voice offered the boy various bits of advice when he was feeling poorly, on one occasion counseling him to "eat plenty of bread and molasses," which cheered him considerably.

In 1838, seeking to improve their lot, the Davis family moved across the Hudson River to Poughkeepsie. Although the change brought only further decline in the family fortunes, it did afford young Andrew a brief exposure to formal education. After a few months, however, the barely literate lad left school to become first a grocery clerk, then an apprentice shoemaker. And that might have been the end of the story had not one J. Stanley Grimes visited Poughkeepsie in the fall of 1843 to lecture on the fascinating new topic of the day, animal magnetism.

Animal magnetism, a term originally coined by the eighteenth-century Austrian physician Franz Anton Mesmer, referred to an impalpable and all-pervasive magnetic fluid that was said to flow through the human body and

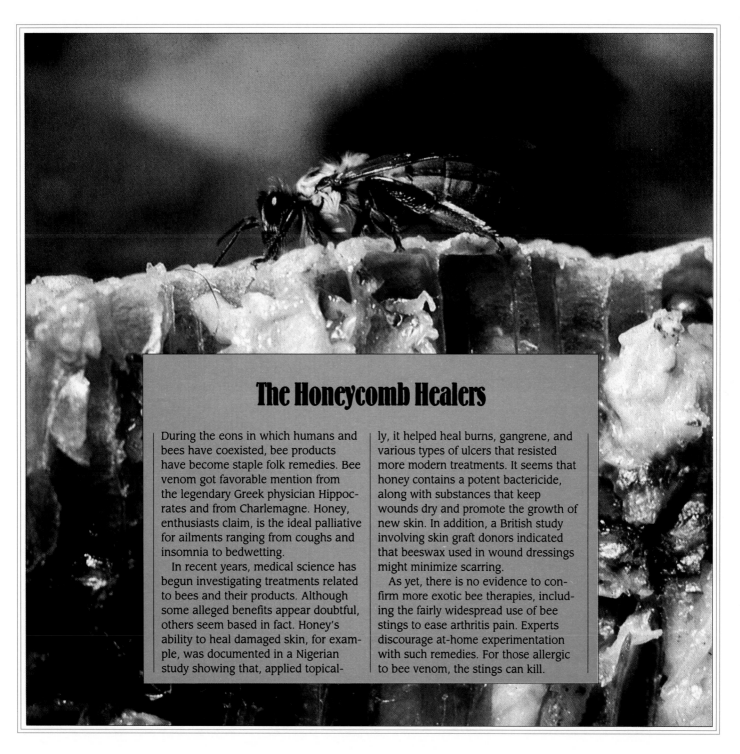

The Honeycomb Healers

During the eons in which humans and bees have coexisted, bee products have become staple folk remedies. Bee venom got favorable mention from the legendary Greek physician Hippocrates and from Charlemagne. Honey, enthusiasts claim, is the ideal palliative for ailments ranging from coughs and insomnia to bedwetting.

In recent years, medical science has begun investigating treatments related to bees and their products. Although some alleged benefits appear doubtful, others seem based in fact. Honey's ability to heal damaged skin, for example, was documented in a Nigerian study showing that, applied topical-

ly, it helped heal burns, gangrene, and various types of ulcers that resisted more modern treatments. It seems that honey contains a potent bactericide, along with substances that keep wounds dry and promote the growth of new skin. In addition, a British study involving skin graft donors indicated that beeswax used in wound dressings might minimize scarring.

As yet, there is no evidence to confirm more exotic bee therapies, including the fairly widespread use of bee stings to ease arthritis pain. Experts discourage at-home experimentation with such remedies. For those allergic to bee venom, the stings can kill.

Medicinal Mix of Old Gods and New

Centuries ago, Africans packed into the holds of slave ships brought with them to the New World one hedge against despair—their religion. It was a highly personal faith in which humans communed directly with their gods and goddesses, who, in turn, intervened regularly in the affairs of men and women. The gods could even inhabit the bodies of worshipers and speak through them. Accessible and ubiquitous, the divinities were wont to behave much as humans did. They could be jealous or loving, malignant or be-

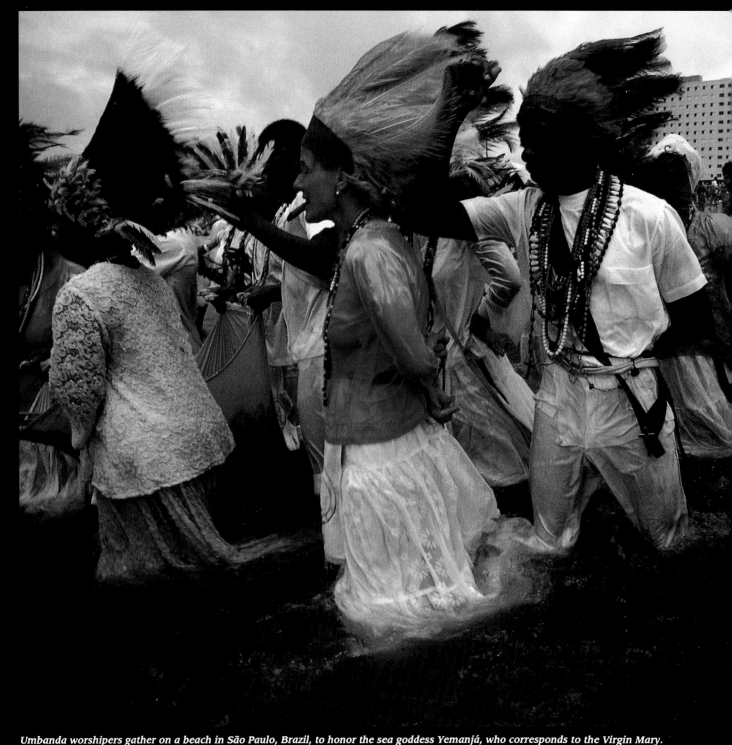

Umbanda worshipers gather on a beach in São Paulo, Brazil, to honor the sea goddess Yemanjá, who corresponds to the Virgin Mary.

nign. They enjoyed human pleasures—good tobacco or a dram of rum—and could be swayed by prayer and flattery and sacrifice. Above all, they were powerful. Properly propitiated, their beneficence was boundless, and healing was among their gifts to bestow.

The Africans clung to their gods but in time had to disguise them. The New World masters ruled that slaves should accept Christianity, usually Catholicism. A merger of gods and saints in new, syncretic religions resulted: Voodoo in Haiti and the American South; Santería in Cuba and Puerto Rico; and in Brazil, Macumba, with its Umbanda and Candomblé sects, which also add Spiritist and native Indian elements. The old gods of some African peoples live on in these religions, which are still practiced today.

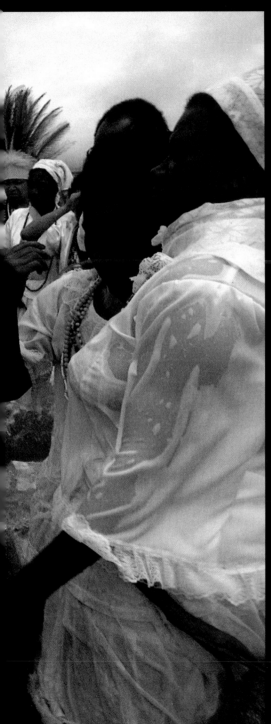

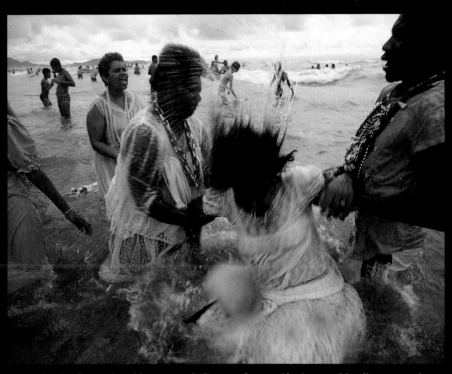

Immersion in the sea is said to assure believers of Yemanjá's love and healing protection.

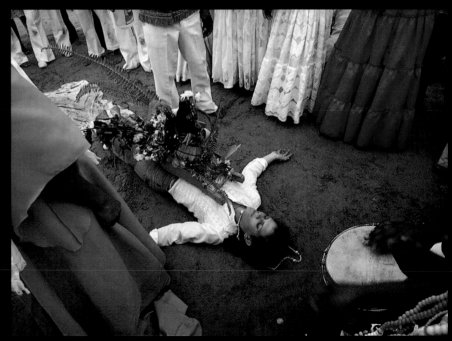

During the rites, mediums surround a flower-strewn patient to attempt a group healing.

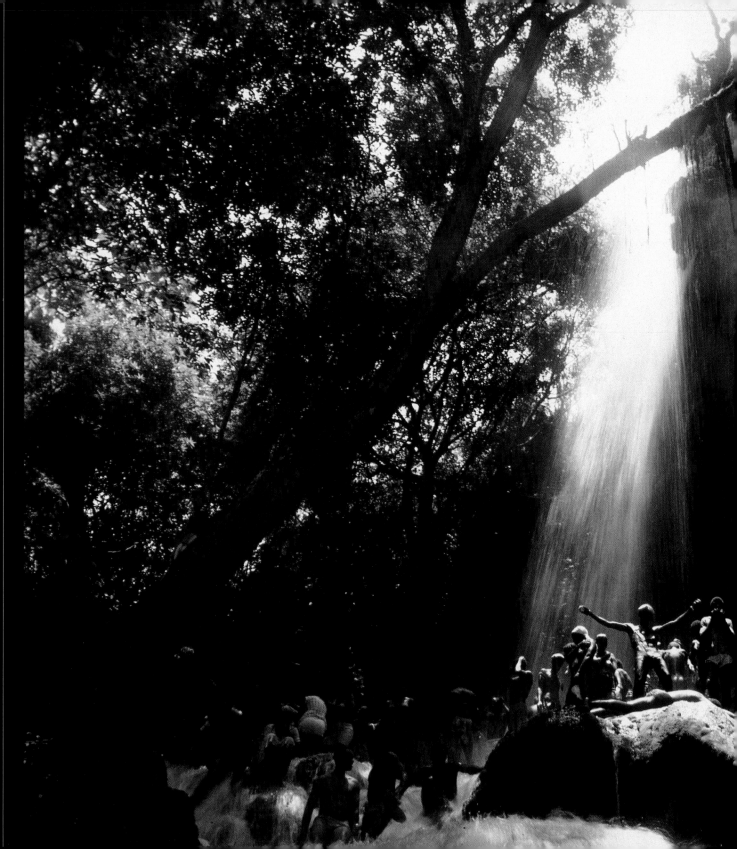

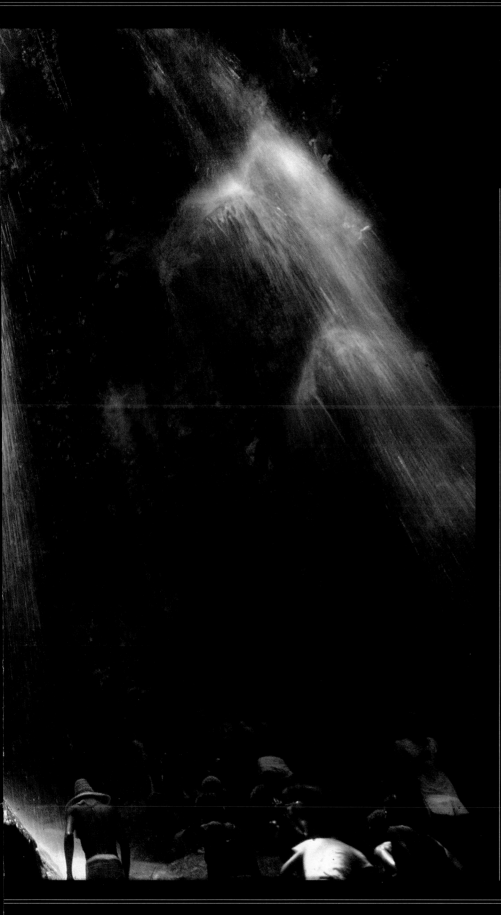

Voodoo abounds with spirits; its name comes from the word *vodun*—"spirit" in the Fon language of West Africa.

Most exalted of the spirits are the *loa,* the gods and goddesses, who correspond to various Christian saints and who rule natural forces, strong emotions, cataclysms: fire, water, earth, love, death, war, and such. There are also spirits of the dead and spirits that dwell in seemingly soulless things—rocks and trees, waterfalls and ponds.

Earth, the source of life, and water, the sustainer of life, are vital in Voodoo, especially in the religion's healing practices. In Haiti, there are festivals each year in which believers seek healing or continued good health at sacred sites of water or mud.

Every July 16, for instance, thousands trek to a shade-dappled glen where the Tombe River cascades over a precipice onto rocks one hundred feet below. It is a holy place called Saut d'Eau, where the Virgin Mary—or, some say, Erzulie Freda, the loa of love—was supposedly sighted twice in the nineteenth century. The waters of Saut d'Eau are said to heal and the pounding falls to strengthen the life force. Erzulie Freda's festival is followed nine days later by a celebration sixty miles north of Saut d'Eau in the village of Plaine du Nord. There, believers immerse themselves in mud, beseeching health from the war god Ogoun Feray or his Christian counterpart, Saint James the Greater.

During the July festival at Saut d'Eau, the Voodoo faithful climb atop a rock to receive the full force of a waterfall whose waters, they say, enhance the life force.

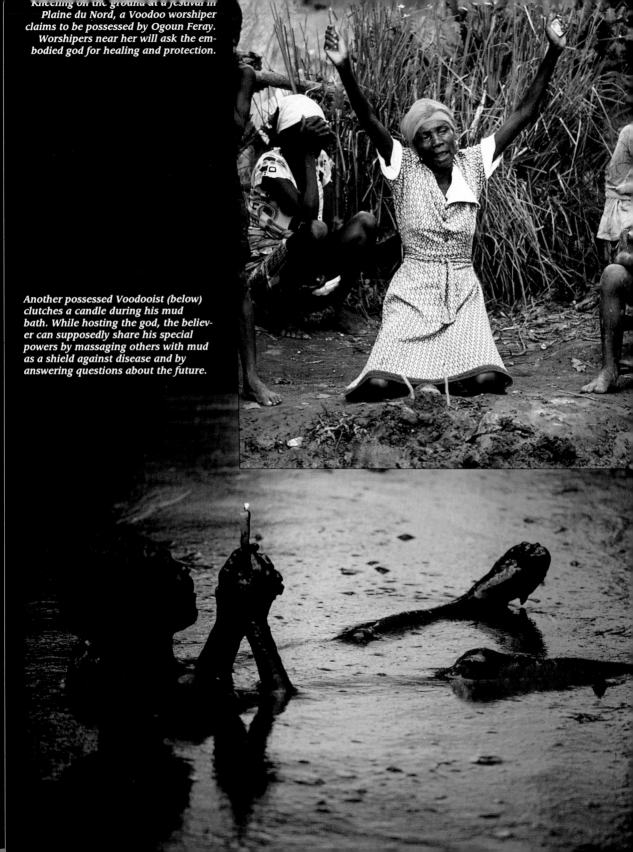

Kneeling on the ground at a festival in Plaine du Nord, a Voodoo worshiper claims to be possessed by Ogoun Feray. Worshipers near her will ask the embodied god for healing and protection.

Another possessed Voodooist (below) clutches a candle during his mud bath. While hosting the god, the believer can supposedly share his special powers by massaging others with mud as a shield against disease and by answering questions about the future.

govern health. "Magnetizers" such as Grimes toured the country claiming to rebalance those fluids that for one reason or another had ceased to flow smoothly, thus creating illness. Their technique usually consisted of putting the patient into a trance, after which the operator passed hands or a wand over the diseased areas, ostensibly to correct the patient's flow and restore him to health and vitality.

Davis, who was in the audience, volunteered as a subject, but Grimes was unable to entrance the young man. Later, however, Davis and a local tailor named William Levingston began practicing on their own, and the tailor succeeded in putting him into a so-called magnetic sleep. Davis allegedly revealed himself a gifted clairvoyant. Not only did he appear to read a newspaper pressed to his forehead and tell the time on pocket watches of persons across the room, he also demonstrated an astonishing talent for medical clairvoyance. He claimed he could correctly diagnose diseases by merely looking at people.

Levingston and Davis recognized a sensational act when they saw it, and for more than a year they performed together, displaying a mix of apparently clairvoyant diagnoses and therapeutics, along with assorted other conventional stage mesmerist skills. To those who found it remarkable that an uneducated cobbler's apprentice could appear so knowledgeable about anatomy and the like, Davis explained that during his trances the human body, indeed all of nature, became transparent. "By looking through space directly into Nature's laboratory, or else into medical establishments, I easily acquired the common (and even the Greek and Latin) names of various medicines, and also of many parts of the human structure, its anatomy, its physiology, its neurology."

One of his patients was a Universalist minister named Gibson Smith, who was quite taken by the seer's diagnostic powers. He claimed that Davis had described "very accurately where a disease with which I had long been afflicted was located—its cause—describing also the pain which I suffered from it and the weakness occasioned by it most perfectly." Smith included this testimonial in a little pamphlet entitled *Clairmativeness,* in which he recorded some of the seventy or eighty clairvoyant medical examinations Davis performed.

In Davis's own 1857 autobiography, *The Magic Staff,* the seer recalled a case typical of those encountered during his years on the healing circuit. A man approached Davis asking to be cured of a hearing loss. The seer entered a trance and while under its influence announced that the nature of the illness "called for the magnetic moisture of the rat." He prescribed placing warm skins of freshly killed rats around each of the man's ears every night for a certain length of time. Of the cure's efficacy Davis reported, "I subsequently heard that the disagreeable remedy wrought his much desired restoration."

Then, at the age of nineteen, Davis reportedly underwent a kind of personal epiphany comparable to those experienced by soon-to-be shamans; he fell into a prolonged somnambulent trance, wandered about for an entire night, then awoke the next morning to find himself in the mountains some forty miles from home. During his trance, he recalled having conversations with Galen, the celebrated Greek physician, and with Emanuel Swedenborg, the eighteenth-century Swedish mystic. Davis had been chosen as a divine oracle, they declared, and his purpose in life was to be the earthly medium for "nature's revelations," which were to be set down on paper so that others might share in the knowledge.

Davis promptly forsook Levingston and their psychic showcase to devote himself to this higher purpose. He moved to New York City, engaged an herbalist named S. Silas Lyon as his new mesmerist and a Universalist minister, the Reverend William Fishbough, to act as his scribe. Davis continued to give clairvoyant diagnoses and treatments to support the trio, but his real work—the dictating of a series of cosmic revelations—began on November 28, 1845. The sessions, 157 in all, spanned fourteen months. On each occasion, Davis would enter the catalyptic trance he had by now learned to self-induce, then speak for periods of up to four

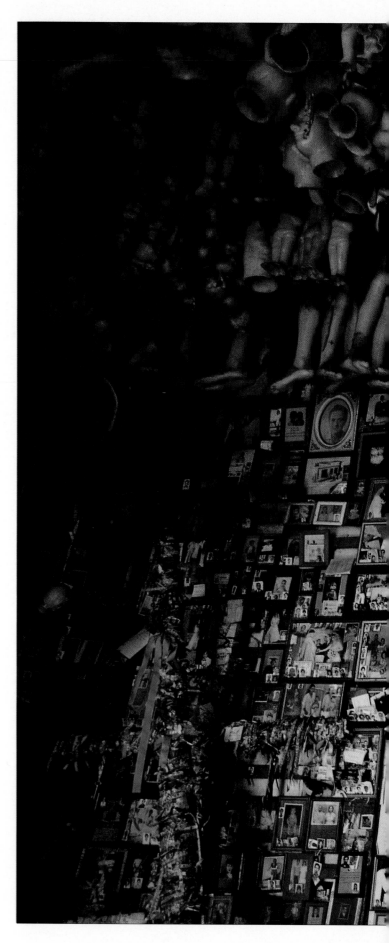

hours on subjects ranging from the "divine Positive Power," which animated all of life, to the creation of the earth and the reform and reorganization of society.

The resulting 782-page tome was published in 1847, under the cumbersome title *The Principles of Nature, Her Divine Revelations, and a Voice to Mankind.* Within weeks of its appearance, however, controversy surrounded the book. Some who initially praised it now pointed out errors in the work. In addition, many ideas and beliefs expressed as Davis's own were apparently derived from those of well-known historians and philosophers, including Swedenborg. But when critics suggested Davis had read those savants' works and simply paraphrased them in his trance, the seer claimed to have read only one book in his life—a romance novel called *The Three Spaniards.*

Whether due to controversy or merit, *Revelations* made Davis famous far beyond the precincts of medicine. It even seemed for a time that he had forsaken healing the individual in favor of healing the world. But eventually, as the profits from his philosophical works began to diminish, Davis resumed his therapeutic activities. He remained a prolific author, however, and in 1861, published a sensible little work entitled *The Harbinger of Health Containing Medical Prescription for the Human Body and Mind.* In that book, Davis set forth the foundation on which he believed health ought to be maintained and restored. He also came remarkably close to expounding twentieth-century theories of holistic medicine.

On the causes of disease, he wrote, "The truth is, that, accidents excepted, *the great majority of human bodily diseases are of mental origin.*" He marveled at "the perfect adaptation and competency of man's vital energies to self-repair and harmonize the bodily organs" and declared that "the whole *Materia Medica*—astringents, tonics, emollients, corrosives, stimulants, sedatives, narcotics, refrigerants, anti-spasmodics, antiseptics, sialagogues, expectorants, emetics, diaphoretics . . . all, yea all, may be found in that wonderful repository of health and disease, the *Constitution of Man!*" Davis thought that the best patients were those

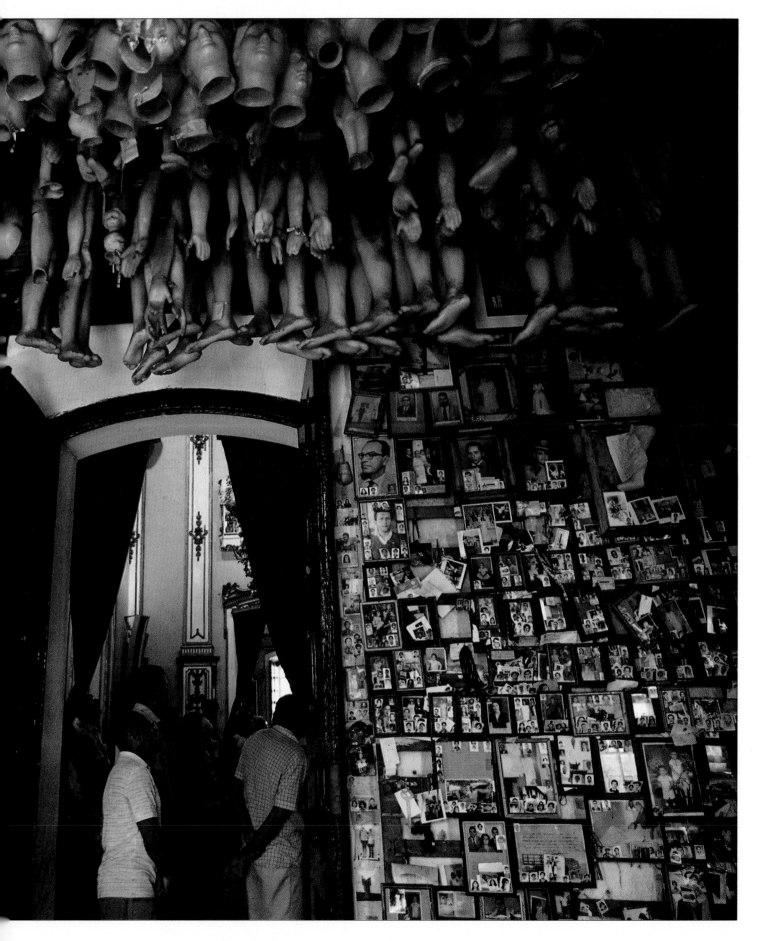

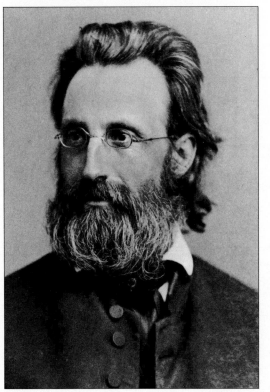

persons of a disciplined mind because they tended to be most responsive to the magnetic energies and probings of the healer, a relationship he described in shamanistic terms. "The brain and body of the operator become one o'ermastering positive power, to which, without resistance, the subject surrenders himself, both physically and mentally. . . . The operator may image his thoughts upon the subject's brain . . . [causing him] to forget his own individuality, and take on the feelings and exhibit the striking characteristics of the operator."

Davis followed his own prescription for living the healthy life "by sleeping and working and living in accordance with the requisites of nature's laws." He died at the venerable age of eighty-four on January 13, 1910.

Nine months after the Poughkeepsie Seer's death, a man who was in many ways Davis's spiritual successor came to national attention in the pages of the *New York Times*. The article was headlined "Illiterate Man Becomes a Doctor When Hypnotized—Strange Power Shown by Edgar Cayce Puzzles Physicians." It went on to tell how Edgar Cayce, a thirty-three-year-old, mild-mannered, somewhat shy country fellow from Kentucky, regularly went into trances in order to diagnose and cure the sick. The newspaper quoted Dr. Wesley H. Ketchum, a reputable physician, graduate of one of the country's leading medical institutions, and a self-avowed skeptic, who had been investigating Cayce in depth for four years. Ketchum was particularly impressed by Cayce's grasp of clinical detail and terminology when in a trance. "His psychological terms and description of the nervous anatomy would do credit to any professor of nervous anatomy. There is no faltering in his speech and all his statements are clear and concise. He handles the

most complex jawbreakers with as much ease as any Boston physician, which to me is quite wonderful, in view of the fact that while in his normal state he is an illiterate man, especially along the line of medicine, surgery or pharmacy."

Not surprisingly, the press, the public, and the medical profession now clamored for every detail of Cayce's life, and the curriculum vitae began tumbling forth. Edgar had been born on March 18, 1877, the only son of a small-time tobacco farmer living in Hopkinsville, Kentucky. Although he would later claim to have had scattered paranormal experiences as a small child, the first clear indications that Cayce had the gift of healing were said to have appeared when he was sixteen years old, in the aftermath of a minor injury on the baseball field.

Young Cayce had been struck at the base of the spine by a pitched ball, and although he sustained no serious injury, he began behaving somewhat strangely. At home that evening the normally docile Edgar stormed about, shouting, laughing uproariously, throwing things, and quarreling with everyone. His father sent him to bed, where the boy soon fell into a profound sleep. As his concerned parents stood over him, a voice seemingly brought up from the depths of Edgar's body commanded Mrs. Cayce to prepare a special poultice and to place it on the back of his head. She did as the mysterious voice requested. The boy then slept normally, and the next morning he arose his old self again, with no apparent recollection of the strange happenings of the previous evening.

Cayce subsequently learned to put himself into a trance, but only occasionally over the next few years did he perform health readings, and then just for friends. At age twenty-one Cayce left home for Louisville, Kentucky, to find work. Soon the young man began suffering severe headaches and sore throats that left him unable to speak above a whisper. He quit his job, moved back home, and began consulting physicians of every sort. After a year of ineffective treatments, Cayce turned for help to a local hypnotist named Al Layne. Significantly, Cayce did not want Layne to hypnotize him—Cayce knew he could induce his own trance; rather, he wanted Layne to act as his conductor once the trance state had been reached. Accordingly, Layne

sat beside the supine Cayce, observing the psychic's breathing. When Cayce appeared fully submerged, Layne instructed him to look at his body, locate the trouble, and describe what he saw. In a few minutes, Cayce began to mumble. Then, in fully audible tones, he said, ''Yes, we can see the body.'' Those six words would become a Cayce trademark in years to come.

Cayce went on to define his speech problem as partial paralysis of the vocal cords triggered by stress. The young man then directed Layne to increase blood circulation to his stricken throat by means of hypnotic suggestion. As Layne spoke, calling forth the healing flow, Cayce's neck flushed a violent red. After twenty minutes, Layne told Cayce to resume normal circulation and to awaken; with that Cayce opened his eyes, sat up, spat out a small amount of blood, and pronounced himself cured.

For the next forty years, the man who became known as the Sleeping Prophet devoted his life to psychic enterprises. Most of his work was centered on healing, but he also gave life readings to clients wishing information on previous incarnations, prophesies on world catastrophes, and dream interpretations.

Hopkinsville soon grew too small for Cayce. After a succession of moves, he received instructions during a reading to relocate in Virginia Beach, Virginia, and moved his operation there in 1926. Contributions rolled in—twenty dollars was the suggested donation for each reading, but many grateful clients sent much more—and his once tiny operation expanded considerably. In time, there was a fully staffed hospital, a foundation for managing finances, and an organization known eventually as the Association for Research and Enlightenment to oversee records of Cayce's cures.

Cayce, for his part, remained a modest, introverted, deeply religious man who stuck close to his family, as

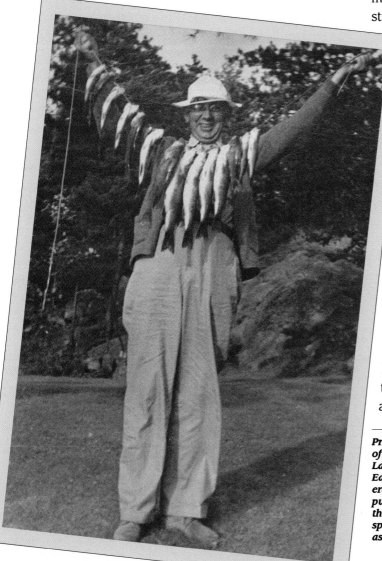

Proudly holding aloft a string of fish just pulled from the St. Lawrence River, a beaming Edgar Cayce poses for the camera in 1939. Such ordinary pursuits were characteristic of the unassuming Cayce, despite his extraordinary career as a trance healer and seer.

well as his vegetable garden, when not acting as healer and clairvoyant. Even when providing readings—usually twice a day, in the morning and afternoon—his technique was typically low-key, with none of the theatrical trappings employed by many self-proclaimed psychics who came before or after him. He would lie on a couch, shirt collar and cuffs loosened, shoes off. He would go quickly into a trance. At his side were usually his wife, Gertrude, who directed the questioning, and his secretary, who recorded Cayce's remarks verbatim. Sometimes the patient would be in the room, but as the healer's fame grew, Cayce began to receive hundreds of written requests for help. For these patients, he set up appointments for absentee readings. With Gertrude supplying the name and address of the patient, Cayce claimed to "see the body" clearly; he required only that the patient be in a cooperative frame of mind and mentally communicate clues about the sickness across the distance. After diagnosing the cause of the illness, Cayce would make a series of recommendations for healing.

He also made a practice of referring some patients to local doctors for continuing therapy; how he came to know spontaneously the names of these doctors, often in towns and cities he had never even visited, was yet another mystery. On one occasion he told a distraught mother from New York City to take her sick child to a certain "Dobbins" when they got home. But when the mother attempted to contact a Dr. Dobbins, she found no such person listed in the telephone book. After further searching, she learned that an osteopath named Frank Dobbins had only just arrived in her borough, which was presumably why his name did not yet appear in the directory.

Another baffling aspect of Cayce's practice involved his drug prescriptions. Often the remedies included formulations that either had been deemed old-fashioned and thus dropped from the current pharmacopoeia or were still in laboratory development and could not possibly be known to anyone but the chemists involved. Sometimes the formulations were just plain odd, such as "calcios," a calcium supple-

ment made from pulverized chicken bones, and "cimex lectularius," the juice of pressed bed bugs, which was recommended for dropsy, phlebitis, and nephritis.

Despite Cayce's large following, or perhaps because of it, his life was dogged by turmoil and controversy. The Depression took its toll on his Association for Research and Enlightment, and the foundation was forced to sell much of its Virginia Beach real estate. The healer also fell afoul of the law from time to time, being charged on various occasions with fortunetelling, violations of the drug laws, and even complicity in a murder—the result of his having correctly identified a killer during a psychic trance. Although Cayce was always found innocent of the charges, the experiences took their toll.

When World War II broke out and Cayce's two grown sons went to fight, he became more engrossed than ever in psychic matters. Letters poured in with desperate pleas for information on the whereabouts of missing servicemen and for help in healing the wounded. Some of his trances were spent in less personal psychic explorations, including those that resulted in his famed, amazingly detailed descriptions of the supposed lost continent of Atlantis. Cayce stepped up the number of his readings until he was spending most of each day in psychic investigations; he collapsed, physically and emotionally exhausted, in August 1944. To treat his own problem, he gave himself a reading and was told to rest "until he is well or dead." Shortly thereafter he suffered a stroke and died on January 3, 1945.

Meanwhile, the Association for Research and Enlightenment had regained its financial strength during the war and now dedicated itself to advancing Cayce's research under the guidance of his heirs. By the late 1980s, the Cayce Foundation boasted one of the largest centers of psychic studies in the world, with approximately 90,000 active members and some 1,500 satellite clinics, camps, and study groups scattered all over the world. The heart of the organization's work, however, was its vast library of more than 14,000 Cayce readings, which have since been painstakingly interpreted and cross-referenced under such head-ings as diseases, remedies, symptoms, and astrological connections. Here, succeeding generations of believers continue to consult the master for medical and spiritual guidance from beyond the grave.

Was Cayce truly psychic? Skeptics point out that patients gave him much information about their diseases and clues to the probable causes in their letters. And the healer's advice, as one critic noted, simply combined "homespun remedies with sound, commonsense recommendations to the patient and his family." Further, the evidence for Cayce's successes is purely anecdotal, based largely on testimonials and letters of thanks. There is little data from physicians or other clinicians to confirm or refute claims of miraculous healing, thus complicating the task of determining whether—or, at the least, to what extent—a genuine psychic factor was involved in Cayce's work.

Whatever the truth of the matter, Cayce was unquestionably the most influential, and perhaps the most gifted, of the modern trance healers. But while Cayce and others claimed to have received their healing powers from some divine force, there existed another group of contemporary healers who believed their revelations came from the spirits of discarnate mortals who had long since passed over. One such spiritual healer was Harry Edwards, who came on the British scene during World War I.

Edwards was not the first to recognize his purported healing abilities. During World War I, he was in charge of a crew of Arabs laying railroad tracks in the Middle East. Accidents were frequent, but the workmen claimed that when Edwards treated their wounds, they healed especially quickly. Edwards brushed off their claims, but the crew continued to call him the *hakim,* or healer. Nevertheless, more than fifteen years would pass before Edwards discovered his talent for himself.

A businessman with an amateur's interest in magic and Spiritualism, Edwards first became intrigued with the possibilities of psychic healing in 1935 while meditating for a friend who was dying of advanced tuberculosis in a dis-

tant hospital. Suddenly, Edwards later recalled, he became aware that his mind's eye had somehow traveled to the hospital and was fixed on a certain bed there. As he continued to meditate, the image of his friend appeared before him and he felt a strange energy passing through him. When he was notified the following day that the friend seemed to be making a spontaneous recovery, it occurred to Edwards that he might have inadvertently taken an astral voyage and become the medium for this seemingly miraculous reversal.

Edwards decided to research the matter further, and in an effort to sharpen his newly discovered skill, he tried working under self-hypnosis, just as Cayce and other contemporary Spiritualist healers had done. But he found that he was able to diagnose and channel spirit messages just as well through meditation alone. Edwards held public demonstrations of his healing talents, and predictably, as his fame grew so did the volume of mail requesting absentee healing. Edwards came to the conclusion that absentee healing worked fully as well as the person-to-person variety, and unlike Cayce, he found no positive correlation between patient cooperation and success; it seemed not to matter one way or the other.

In his heyday, Edwards is said to have received some 2,000 letters daily at his Healing Sanctuary, a country mansion in Surrey, England. According to his own records, the healer averaged an 80 to 90 percent recovery rate on those patients selected for treatment, although strict scientific accounting to support such claims was never made.

Asked to define the source of his medical information, Edwards always described himself as merely the "attuned receiver *through whom* the spirit healing forces are received for transmission to the patient." Those forces varied, he explained, but two nineteenth-century giants, the French chemist Louis Pasteur and the English surgeon Lord Joseph Lister, were cited as among his spirit doctors. According to one source, a review of a large number of Edwards's cases turned up no cures that could not be explained as psychogenic—that is, taking place only in the mind—or as the

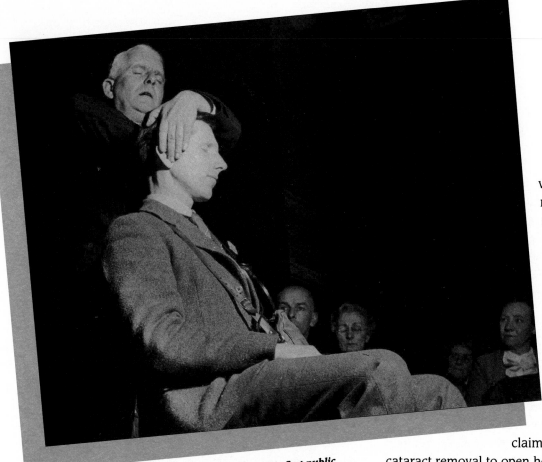

Harry Edwards lays his hands on a patient at his first public healing demonstration, held in London in 1947. He downplayed his alleged gift, saying, "I myself have never cured anyone. My part is simply that of a channel for the healing powers."

who died in 1937. Once Chapman realized the identity of his spirit guide, he took up healing as his life's work. The enthusiastic medium even went so far as to buy the good doctor's former home and office—the logical place from which to conduct his spirit practice—in the town of Aylesbury, just north of London.

George Chapman describes the technique he uses as "etheric surgery," and he claims to carry out everything from cataract removal to open heart surgery without so much as touching the patient. Chapman believes that he and Lang are able to do this because they treat the etheric body, a field of energy that is said to exist in correspondence with the physical body.

Chapman has inspired numerous books and articles in which satisfied patients describe the experience of going to "Dr. Lang's" office. Probably the most extensive documentation is to be found in J. Bernard Hutton's 1966 book, *Healing Hands.* The author, whose other works cover such subjects as the supernatural and espionage, became aware of Chapman's work when he himself suffered a loss of eyesight as a result of a serious illness. At the urging of his wife, Hutton made an appointment with "Dr. Lang." Initially skeptical, the author received what he considered a miraculous cure at the hands of the entranced medium. Deciding to investigate Chapman further, Hutton interviewed many of his patients and checked medical records in an effort to determine "the authenticity and credibility of Lang's and Chapman's achievements." Most of the patients he interviewed described experiences similar to his own.

From the moment the patient arrives at the office, no mention is made of Chapman, only of "the doctor." And in the treatment room, patients are greeted by what appears

result of spontaneous remission. The public, however, continued to be enthralled, and when Edwards died in 1976, two of his colleagues, who were evidently also "attuned," continued his work.

Although Edwards credited his healing successes to the influence of spirit guides, he did not claim to *become* any particular physician during a healing session. That was not the case with another well-known British healer, George Chapman.

A former firefighter from Liverpool, Chapman supposedly discovered his healing powers when he turned to Spiritualism in 1945. It was shortly after the death of his baby daughter, and the grieving Chapman was seeking evidence of life after death. He entered a trance state and, while hypnotized, claimed to have received messages from such diverse healers as an American Indian medicine man and a Chinese surgeon named Chang. Soon after, another, more impressive spirit reportedly presented itself—that of Dr. William Lang, the noted British opthalmologist and surgeon

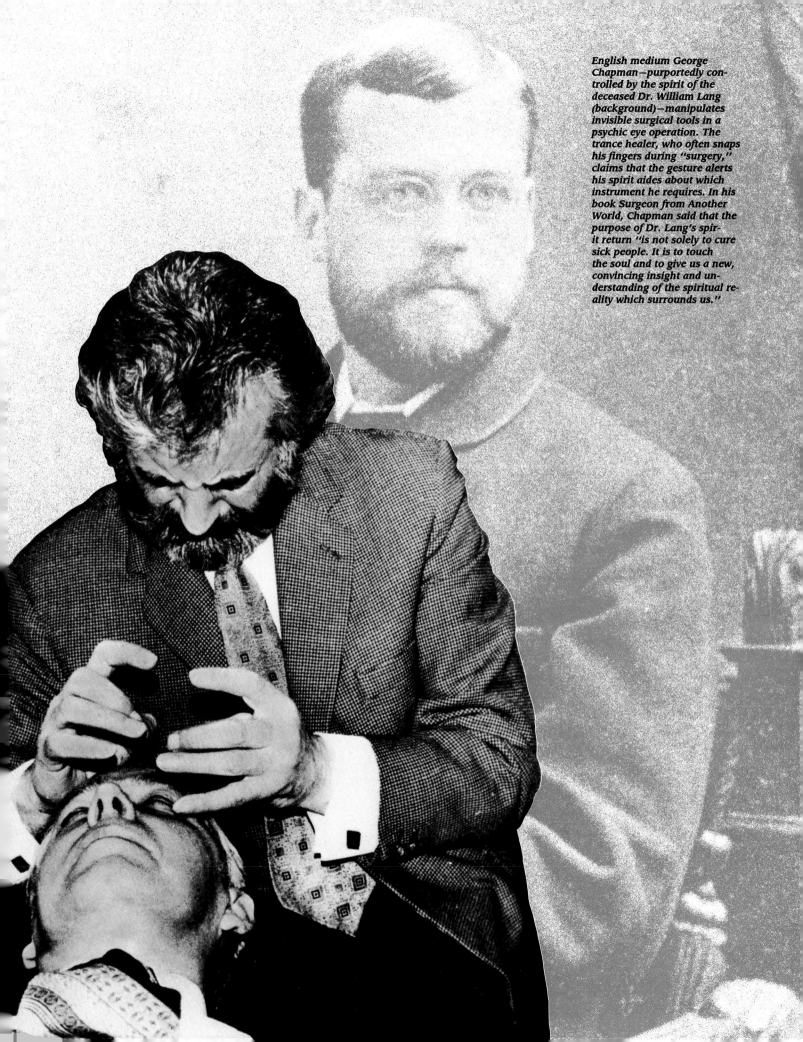

English medium George Chapman—purportedly controlled by the spirit of the deceased Dr. William Lang (background)—manipulates invisible surgical tools in a psychic eye operation. The trance healer, who often snaps his fingers during "surgery," claims that the gesture alerts his spirit aides about which instrument he requires. In his book Surgeon from Another World, Chapman said that the purpose of Dr. Lang's spirit return "is not solely to cure sick people. It is to touch the soul and to give us a new, convincing insight and understanding of the spiritual reality which surrounds us."

to be a stoop-shouldered, quavery-voiced, elderly man. (Dr. Lang was eighty-four years old when he passed away.) As Bernard Hutton recalled, "I could see the resemblance between the standing figure and the photograph of Chapman. But the face—it looked so much older. The wrinkles and lines were marks of true old age, but I knew Chapman was in his forties."

Most of the time Chapman's eyes are tightly closed; he goes into a trance at the start of each day and remains entranced until the last patient of the day has been seen. Acting as Dr. Lang, Chapman talks to the patients, diagnoses their illnesses, and if necessary operates on them with his invisible instruments. A friend or family member accompanying the patient is frequently permitted to observe treatment; in Hutton's interviews these witnesses confirmed that no physicians' tools were ever visible in the office. The patients who underwent "surgery," however, reported experiencing the feeling of the slight twinge of a scalpel being inserted, the prick of a needle, the drawing together of flesh when surgical wounds were closed, and even mild postoperative pain the next day.

Whatever the explanation for Chapman's etheric surgery, it appears to be carried out in a benign and comforting atmosphere by a person who believes in what he is doing. Nevertheless, it seems only a short jump from Chapman's brand of healing to that practiced by the notorious psychic surgeons who flourish in some Third World countries. These alleged miracle workers, who maintain that they are under the spiritual guidance of Jesus Christ or some other great healer, profess to cure by entering their patients' bodies without benefit of an incision and removing dead or diseased tissue. And the great pools of blood and the masses of tumorous material that they bring forth during an operation seem at first glance to confirm the truth of their statements.

But lengthy investigations by William Nolen, a respected American surgeon who underwent psychic surgery, and David Hoy, a Kentucky magician and professional psychic, have shown that actual cutting almost never takes place. Rather, the so-called surgeons practice clever sleight-of-hand tricks, palming pouches of animal blood and odd bits of tissuelike material in their hands, to reveal them at the climactic moment.

Clumsy as the tricks may be, seeing is often believing for people who are desperately sick. And this is the professed aim of many psychic surgeons—to restore health via the placebo effect. They instruct new recruits in their deceptive ways in order to continue what they consider an age-old tradition—healing through faith.

Psychic surgeons enjoy great popularity in Brazil and in the Philippines, where scores of practitioners are estimated to be operating in remote parts of the country. Not only do these putative healers attract thousands of their compatriots, but thanks to a considerable amount of publicity abroad, they draw plane loads of foreigners every month. Most patients are ordinary folk, coping with terminal conditions and desperate to stay alive. Usually their sad stories never come to public attention; but the poignant plight of one American, popular young comic and television star Andy Kaufman, was reported in *Discover* magazine in August 1984 by Martin Gardner, a science writer who specializes in exposing psychic frauds.

According to Gardner, Kaufman had chanced to see a film called *Psychic Phenomena: Exploring the Unknown* in the late 1970s. The film had briefly touched on the work of Philippine psychic surgeons, with only the mildest of disclaimers as to their genuine efficacy. Several years later, in the spring of 1984, Kaufman was told that he was dying of lung cancer; he decided to seek out one of these healers in a last-ditch effort to find a cure. Kaufman went to the clinic of one Ramon "Junior" Labo.

The young actor attended healing sessions twice a day for several days. On each occasion, Labo went through a certain amount of laying on of hands, "balancing of magnetic forces," and massaging with divinely sanctioned oils, while awaiting spiritual guidance. Then, upon receiving what was said to be divine instruction, Labo appeared to pull open Kaufman's diseased chest, staunch a great quantity of blood, and then remove the offending material. A few days later the actor returned to Los Angeles, convinced that the cancer had been eradicated, but in only two months Kaufman was dead. Hospital x-rays indicated that no surgery had ever been performed and that the cancer had proceeded unchecked along its deadly course.

In the face of such contradictory evidence, what case can be made, then, for trance healing? The evidence to date suggests that spirit healers can indeed ease pain, drive away disease, cause the lame to walk and the blind to see— but only some of the time, and not for reasons that can unquestionably be called paranormal or miraculous or divinely inspired. Apparently all healers succeed when they do because perhaps 80 percent of all diseases are either psychogenic or self-limiting and because the human body is naturally inclined to healing both kinds of afflictions when given half a chance. In such a case, the most effective treatment is whatever the patient is most likely to believe in—whether it is the dramaturgy of the shaman, the religious ecstasy of the Christian mystic, or the silent persuasion of the all-knowing physician-scientist—and that is largely a matter of one's culture and personal circumstance.

But what of the other 20 percent of diseases, those

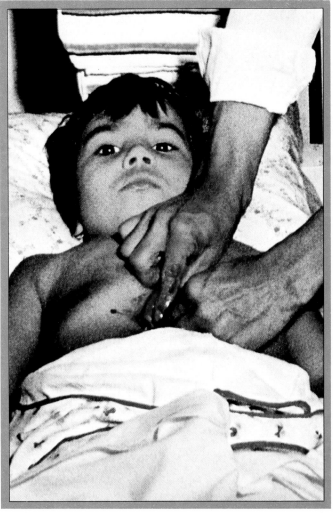

that are physical in origin and do not tend to cure themselves? There is, to date, no convincing scientific evidence to show that illnesses such as malignant cancers, blood diseases, or severe viral or bacterial infections can be permanently cured by any form of alternative, non-medical healing. The intervention of a healer may address some of the symptoms, however. Alleviating pain, reducing anxiety, relieving psychological depression—all seem positive benefits that give the patient and his loved ones the sense that the underlying disease is in retreat. The empowered patient can then call upon his own inner resources to help battle the enemy within.

Such a positive, can-do attitude would likely be applauded by any physician treating a seriously ill patient. Yet the battle rages on between alternative healing and scientific medicine, and it is the patient who is caught squarely in the middle. Critics contend that sufferers who consult alternative therapists before seeking the medical advice of a physician run the risk of masking important symptoms and delaying life-saving treatments. Perhaps the most prudent advice in such a dilemma is offered by the example of Norman Cousins—take an active role in your own health and examine the healing options. Then decide for yourself whether or not to use them—not as a substitute for orthodox medical treatment, but in partnership with it.

Renaissance in Folk Remedies

Long before medicine became a science and drugs were created in test tubes, folk healers employed an extensive—and sometimes bizarre—array of natural pharmaceuticals and techniques to treat the sick. In ancient Mexico, Aztecs plunged their hands deep into anthills to relieve crippling arthritic pain. In colonial New England, the skin of a black cat wrapped around the neck was thought to cure a sore throat. And even today, in eastern Czechoslovakia, people try to banish headaches by wrapping horseradish leaves around their heads.

Although the efficacy of some folk remedies is questionable at best, there exists a great trove of natural healing agents whose effectiveness is supported by modern science. Ancient Egyptians, for example, prescribed castor oil as a laxative and treated heart ailments with the juice of a Mediterranean sea onion, now recognized as one of the strongest known cardiac stimulants. And American Indians used willow bark to relieve the pain of rheumatism long before the advent of aspirin—whose active ingredient is related to a chemical contained in willow bark. Today more than 40 percent of all prescription drugs sold in the United States contain ingredients derived from herbs, plants, and other natural sources. Many of these drugs are based on traditional cures.

No wonder then that in recent times folk medicine has experienced a renaissance of sorts. Physicians and scientists, as well as individuals who are seeking relief from their own maladies, are examining ancient therapies in search of successful cures. Many look for answers in cultures still practicing folk medicine, studying healing methods that are currently in use, such as those presented on the following pages.

Seeking to ease her headache with the aroma of nicotine, Remedios Moya of Valencia, New Mexico, wears cigarette package revenue stamps on her nose. Many cultures believe tobacco has potent curative powers.

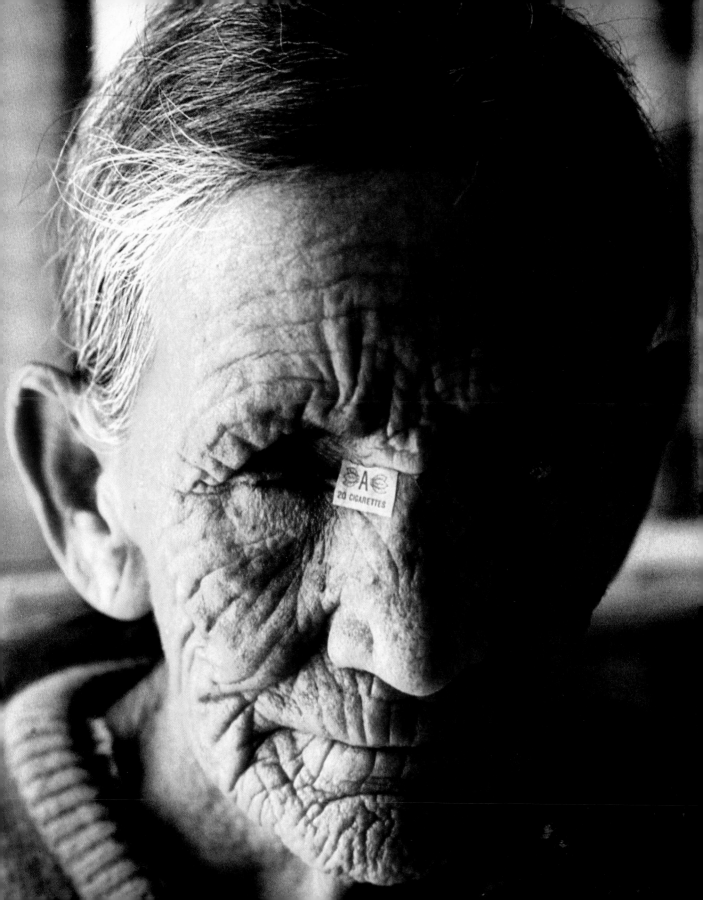

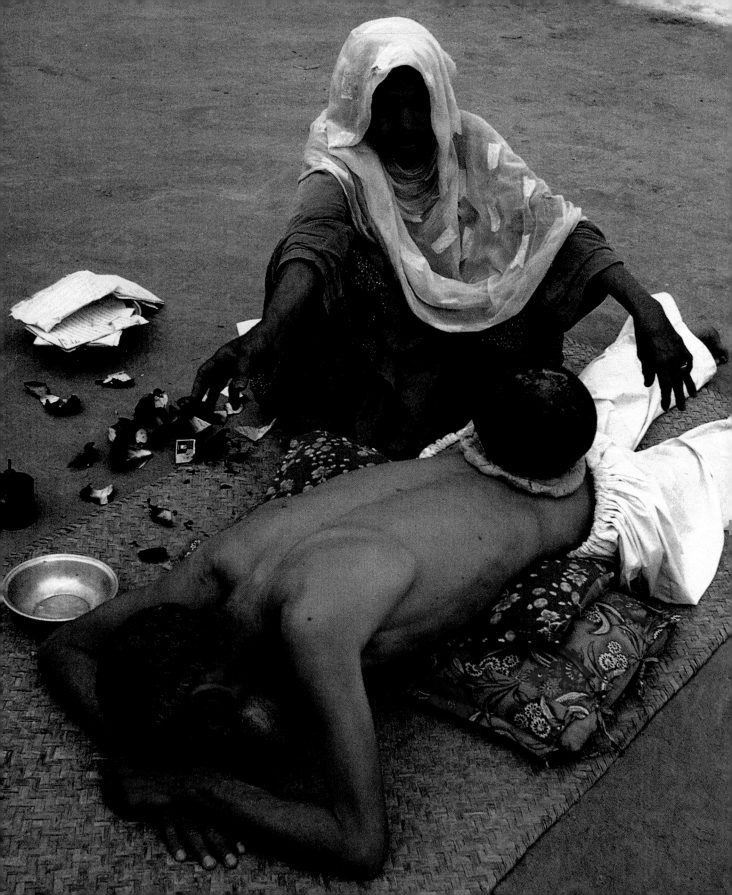

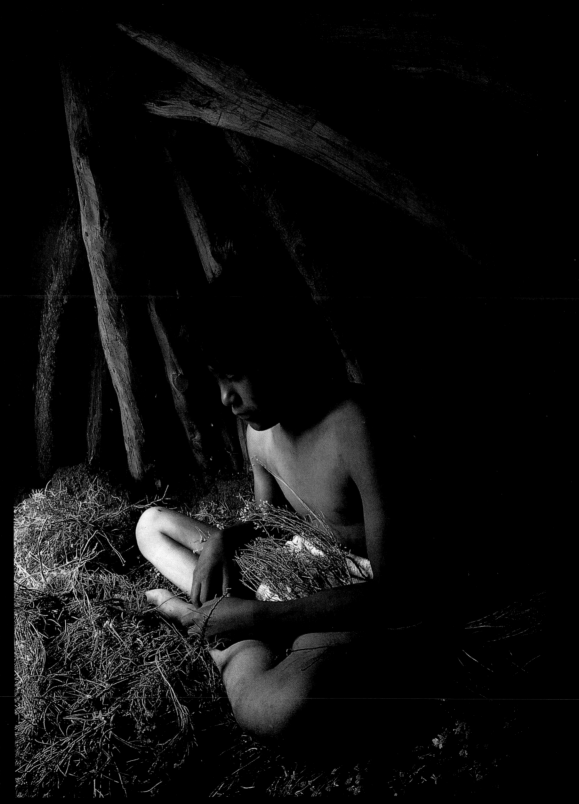

A midwife and healer (left) in a remote, mountainous region of Pakistan ministers to a villager's aching back using bread dough and a bowl. She first places a circle of dough over the painful spot, then deposits bits of paper inscribed with Koranic verses into a clay bowl, sets the paper on fire, and then inverts the bowl on the dough. This procedure produces a moist heat treatment, similar to a poultice.

A Navajo Indian boy (right) suffering from a bad cold waits in a sweat house while a steam bath is readied to ease his discomfort. Heated rocks will be splashed with water and covered with herbs to create a medicinal vapor intended to relieve congestion. The Navajo, who live in the southwestern United States, believe sickness occurs when an individual is not in harmony with himself or with nature and thus, against his will, violates tribal taboos. Herbs and ritual ceremonies are believed to restore harmony.

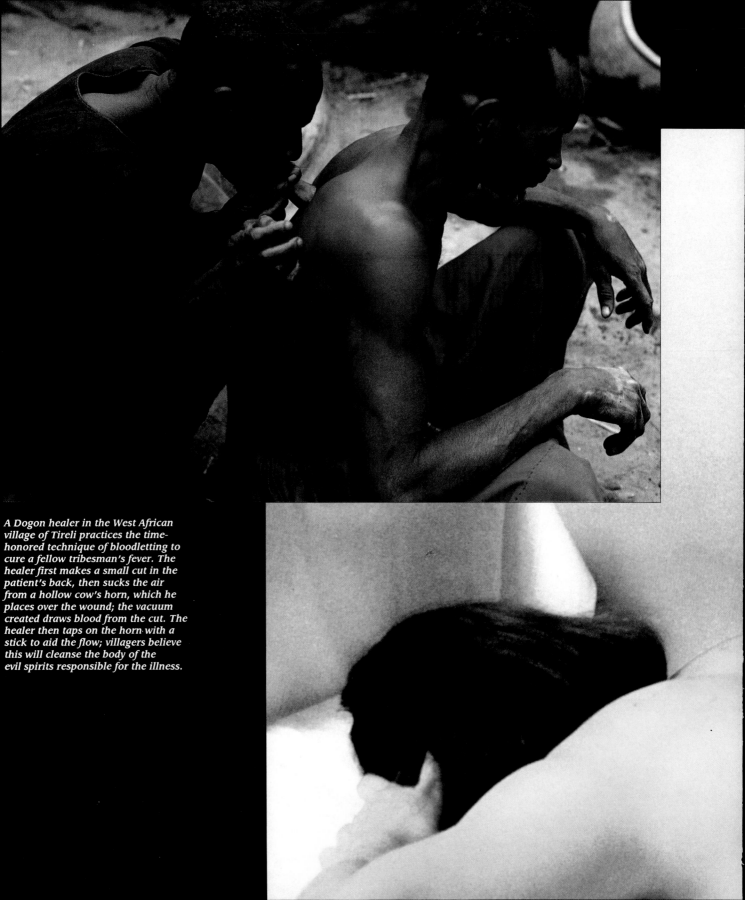

A Dogon healer in the West African village of Tireli practices the time-honored technique of bloodletting to cure a fellow tribesman's fever. The healer first makes a small cut in the patient's back, then sucks the air from a hollow cow's horn, which he places over the wound; the vacuum created draws blood from the cut. The healer then taps on the horn with a stick to aid the flow; villagers believe this will cleanse the body of the evil spirits responsible for the illness.

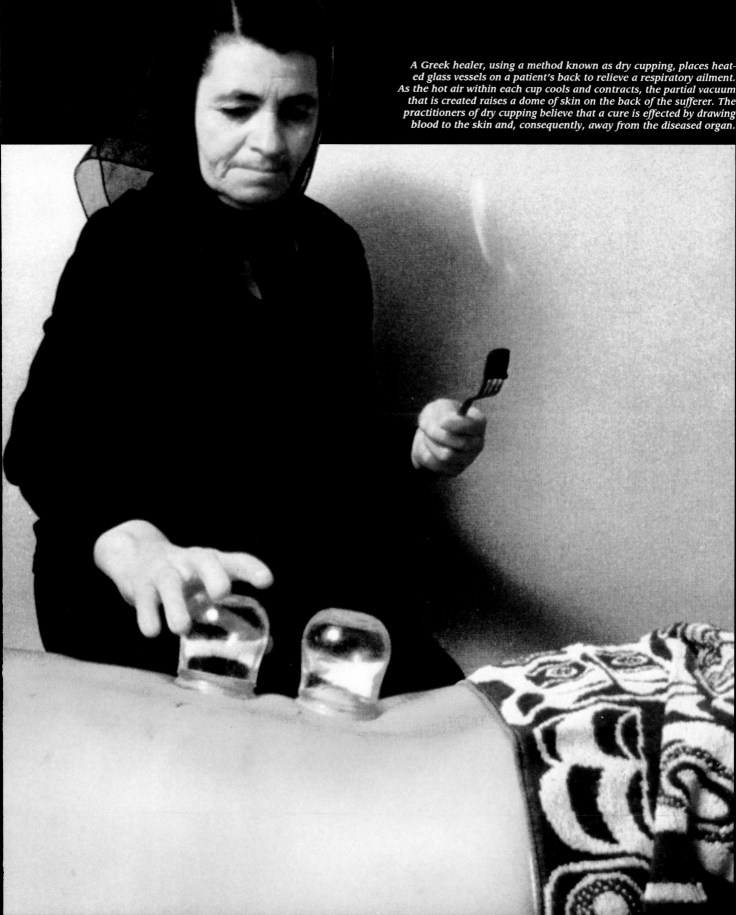

A Greek healer, using a method known as dry cupping, places heated glass vessels on a patient's back to relieve a respiratory ailment. As the hot air within each cup cools and contracts, the partial vacuum that is created raises a dome of skin on the back of the sufferer. The practitioners of dry cupping believe that a cure is effected by drawing blood to the skin and, consequently, away from the diseased organ.

CHAPTER 2

Ancient Arts from the East

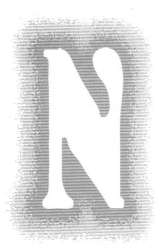

ew York City's hellish South Bronx is a place where many people know about needles—the kind that inject small jolts of death into their veins, day in, day out. Cozet Parker was one of those people, a veteran of needles: a heroin addict and the young mother of an infant who was born a heroin addict. But as she sat in the crowded clinic of the South Bronx's Lincoln Hospital one day in the late 1980s, Cozet Parker was learning about another kind of needle—a half-inch-long, stainless-steel barb, eight of which protruded from strategic points on her ears like pins in a pincushion.

Far from being killers, these needles were supposed to help heal her addiction. The treatment looked painful, but Parker reported that, on the contrary, it made her feel relaxed. Once the hair-thin needles were removed, she said, "I don't get any cravings. I don't think about getting high."

It remains to be seen whether the new needles will permanently wean Parker from the old. But physicians familiar with the treatment contend that it offers real hope, not only for patients in thrall to heroin, but for those addicted to numerous other drugs, notably alcohol and crack—the smokable, powerfully addictive form of cocaine. "I'd say it's the most promising treatment I've seen in fifteen years," says Dr. Bernard Bihari, who oversees the therapy at Kings County Hospital in Brooklyn.

This promising "new" treatment is, of course, acupuncture—one of the oldest therapies known to the healing arts. Chinese physicians have been practicing it for at least 2,500 years and consider it a wide-spectrum weapon against many of the ailments that beset the human race.

Acupuncture is probably the best known of several Eastern therapies that have migrated westward in recent years. In the West, all generally come under the rubric "alternative healing"—a mildly derogatory term that reflects the skepticism these ancient methods encounter among many practitioners of occidental medicine. The doubt seems to be eroding somewhat as more Western doctors display a willingness to study, if not embrace, the old and foreign ways—hoping, perhaps, that a meeting of East and West might yield some useful hybrid. However, if such a merger is to take place, a vast chasm must be crossed, for Eastern and Western healing methods differ not only in technique, but in the deepest philosophical sense.

Put in the simplest way, Western medicine treats dysfunction and disease; Eastern healing treats people. In the West, a patient is generally viewed as a body, a biological organism that is subject to damaging mishaps and to invasion by harmful outside agents. The central concern of occidental healing is to repair damage or to diagnose, isolate, and treat the invading disease. In the East, however, the patient is not merely a body, but an integral amalgam of body, mind, and spirit, all equally important, all interacting constantly—and, at their best, harmoniously—with an environment. This view, reflected in the West in the increasingly popular notion of "holistic health," lies at the root of all the Eastern therapies.

The oldest Eastern healing traditions (and the ones most in vogue today in America and other Western nations) are native to China and India and are rooted in the dominant philosophical systems and ancient religions of those countries—Taoism in China and Hinduism in India. Over the centuries, Chinese and Indian traditions influenced each other, and both impinged greatly on the medical thought and methodology of Japan, Korea, Indonesia, Tibet, Persia, and Southeast Asia.

Holistic healing traditions vary significantly from country to country. But all of them have a common substratum, a way of looking at the world in which health depends not on a discrete science of healing, but on an integral totality in which habits, behavior, and even moral attitudes figure in the well-being of an individual. This view is perhaps best embodied in the ancient Chinese philosophy called Taoism.

According to the Tao (the word means "the Way"—the creative principle that orders the cosmos), the universe is forever in flux, creating and re-creating itself in a complex interplay of energies and potentialities. Always changing, the cosmos is, nevertheless, always ordered. Change is

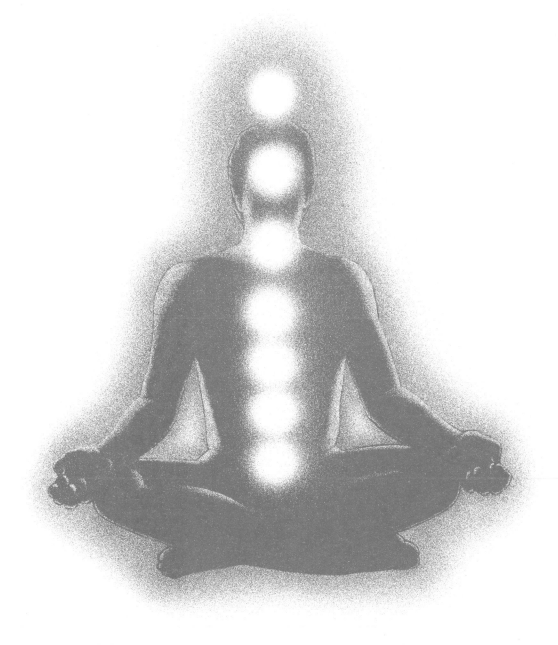

harmonious, an entwining of contending energies that form an inevitable unity. This idea is pictured in a symbol that has become familiar to many Westerners: the joined twin embryos of the yin-yang. Yin and yang represent the apparent opposites that interact to make up the cosmic whole—light and dark, male and female, heaven and earth, for example. In fact, according to the Tao, these forces are not really antithetical, but complementary—different aspects of an essential unity. Each needs the other, and each carries the seed of the other. Yin and yang flow together in a rhythmic and endless dance that expresses the harmony of the cosmos.

These Taoist concepts are essential to understanding Eastern healing because, for followers of this path, the human being is the microcosm of the universe, composed of the same contending universal energies, subject to the same laws. In a state of health, the individual's mind, body, and spirit reflect the blending of the yin-yang: All is in balance, and the total working is harmonious. However, when someone strays from the Way, acting against the flow of nature and the cosmic plan, problems arise—not as a consequence of sin, in the Western sense, but as the ineluctable result of being out of step with the greater whole. Bodily balance between yin and yang can be disturbed, either by immoderation—too much or too little of any one factor—or by blockage of the flow of vital energy that connects and nourishes the various parts. When this happens, the healer's task is to help the individual reestablish the body's attunement to the cosmic scheme. As concepts, the oriental healer

would find the terms *health* and *disease* much less meaningful than *harmony* and *disharmony*.

And harmony is the natural state of things. Physicians of ancient China—unlike their Western counterparts—were paid only when the patient was healthy. Payments ceased with the onset of disease. Not only did this system reinforce the idea that harmony equals good health, it also gave physicians added incentive to get people well quickly and keep them well. For modern practitioners of the oriental ways, the doctor's duty remains to help foster the patient's interdependent mental, physical, and spiritual harmony. The focus is not primarily on curing disease, but on keeping patients free of it. Needless to say, this approach differs considerably from the main thrust of traditional Western medicine.

There is no simple and concise explanation for why Western healing developed along mechanistic, nonmetaphysical lines while its Eastern counterpart held fast to its religious and philosophical origins. But one factor is telling: Much of Western medicine is based on a knowledge of human anatomy derived primarily from surgery and dissection—the direct observation of all the body's inner constituents. In both China and India, however, dissection of human bodies was forbidden for centuries. In China, cutting open a human cadaver was deemed a gross in-

This seventeenth-century wooden figure taught aspiring Chinese physicians the body's meridian routes, the unseen pathways believed to circulate life-giving energy, or qi. At points where meridians branch into channels leading to the skin's surface, acupuncture needles are inserted to regulate qi and to relieve illness.

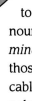

This symbol, purportedly created by the father of classical Chinese medicine, Emperor Fu Xi, in about 3000 BC, shows the forces of yin (dark) and yang (light). The forces are perfectly balanced here, each having the germ of its opposite; any upset in the balance leads to illness.

sult to the dead person's ancestors, and it was not until the eighteenth century that the Chinese began anatomical studies. Moreover, in both China and India, internal surgery was performed sparingly and only as a last resort. What knowledge there was of anatomy came mainly from animal models and from treating centuries of war wounds. Along with this knowledge, Eastern medicine relied on precise observations of the external evidence of internal workings—and on metaphysical beliefs concerning the human being as a reflection of a greater cosmic order.

So it was that in Chinese healing, for instance, there came to be six "solid," or yin, organs (the heart, lungs, liver, kidney, spleen, and "heart protector," or pericardium) that balanced six "hollow," or yang, organs (the small intestine, large intestine, gall bladder, bladder, stomach, and a "triple warmer"—a collective name for what the ancients perceived as three metabolic centers within the body's trunk). Moreover, each organ was thought to be dominated by one of the five elements, or phases of energy, that compose all matter and figure in the universal harmony: fire, wood, earth, metal, and water. Working from what they saw as immutable, predictable patterns that these elements expressed in nature, traditional Chinese doctors extrapolated the functions of the human body, which must, they reasoned, adhere to the same patterns.

But what was the dynamism that animated the body? Oriental healing answered this question with the concept that behind all phenomena was an invisible life force that animated the universe and individuals alike. In humans, its energy flowed through the body, mind, and spirit to vitalize them and regulate their interworkings. For practitioners of Chinese therapies, then and now, the mysterious force is known as *ch'i—qi* in China's modern Pinyin transliteration system. This potent cosmic energy suffuses the body through an invisible network of branching channels called meridians.

The meridian network is likened to irrigation channels that feed and nourish the body and mind—or *body-mind* as it is sometimes written by those wishing to emphasize the inextricable link between the two. The channels supposedly connect the exterior of the body to the interior and link all the fundamental organs to one another. Keeping the meridians unblocked so qi can flow freely is essential to the Chinese notion of health. Correctly distributed, qi is said to provide resistance to disease. A disruption or imbalance in its flow results in illness.

Generally it is said that there are twelve "regular" channels, or primary meridians, all terminating in the toes or fingers. Each is associated with a particular internal organ and is referred to by the organ's name—the heart meridian, liver meridian, and so on. In addition, there are eight "extra," or "extraordinary," channels and many minor connecting ones. Along these channels, like pearls on a string, are the 365 acupuncture points of classical Chinese theory—spots where the meridians, and thus the flow of qi, can be manipulated. The number of presumed acupoints has increased by at least 40 since the founding of the People's Republic of China in 1949. With government funding, researchers located the additional points by using modern equipment that measures the skin's galvanic response to a slight electromagnetic current. Supposedly, the electric probing elicits a more active response at the acupoints than it does elsewhere along the skin.

Acupuncture therapy uses the meridian network as the basis of treatment. A therapeutic needle need not nec-

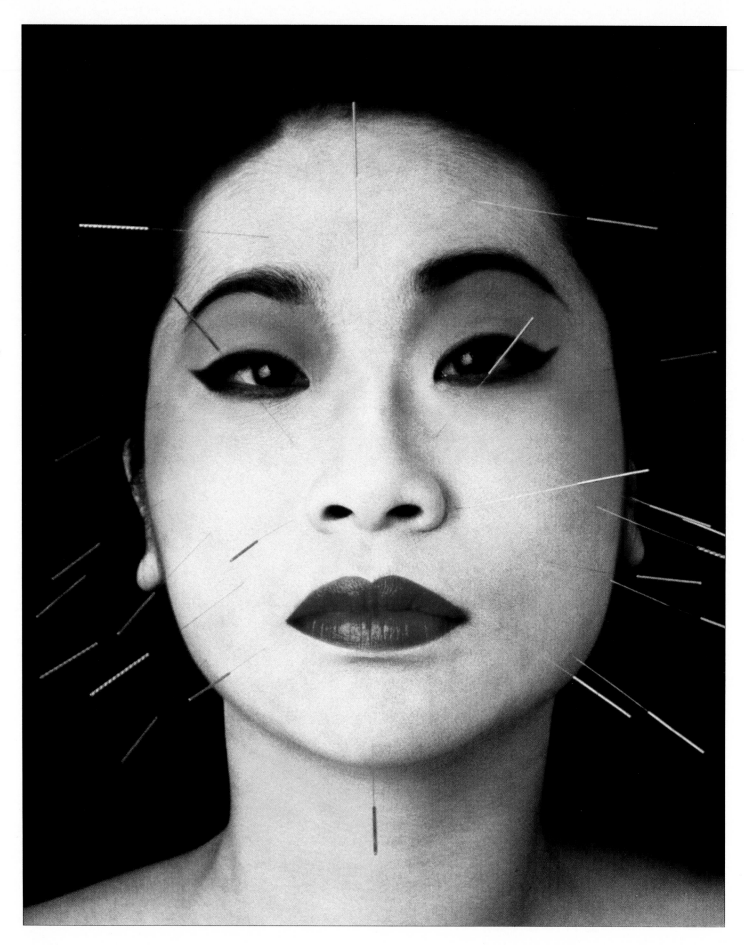

essarily be inserted at the point of presumed blockage or imbalance. Rather, the desired effect can be achieved by using an acupoint known to govern or connect with the body part needing relief. For example, a needle inserted in the toe at the start of the spleen meridian can be felt along all twenty other points of that meridian, points running up the leg and across the hip, abdomen, and chest to the armpit. Thus one needle can affect any one of several areas, some far distant from the point of insertion.

In theory, acupuncture can stimulate the flow of qi or drain off excess. The physician relies on the patient's symptoms to determine which process is needed and precisely how it should be performed. To administer treatment, the practitioner needs a thorough knowledge of the meridian network itself and an understanding of how it reflects the underlying principles of Chinese healing, along with an expert hand in inserting needles correctly and painlessly. The size of the needles used, how deeply they are inserted, how long they should be left in place, and how they should be twirled or otherwise manipulated are all factors that affect the treatment.

There are several adjunct therapies that go along with acupuncture. One of the most popular and venerable of these—just as old as acupuncture itself—is moxibus-

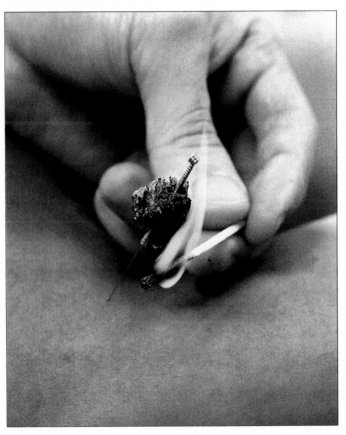

Using a technique called moxibustion to treat a patient's cold, a healer ignites a plug of the herb mugwort, or moxa. The smoldering herb is held above an acupoint or placed atop an acupuncture needle, as here, in order to increase the stimulation of qi.

tion. This procedure also uses meridians and acupoints. A powdered plant substance called moxa (a variety of mugwort) may be attached to the acupuncture needle or shaped into a mound that is placed atop some shielding substance, usually ginger, and applied to the patient's skin at the appropriate acupoint. The plant is then burned, causing heat to penetrate through the shield to the point. More commonly, moxa is rolled into sticks that look like cigars. The lighted tip of the stick is brought close to the skin to create the requisite heating of the acupoint.

Modern therapists sometimes replace the traditional needles with other stimuli. For example, there are electro-acupuncture, which uses a slight electric current; ultrasonography, which employs ultrasonic waves; and laser puncture, which features minute laser beams. Related techniques include acupressure, the application of hand or finger pressure over acupoints, and homeo-acupuncture, the injection of homeopathic solutions into acupoints.

In Chinese tradition, acupuncture claims a long and successful clinical history in dealing with an amazing variety of diseases and disorders. Its alleged flexibility and range rest basically with the underlying notion of qi: Qi is the source of health, and acupuncture regulates qi; therefore, acupuncture can restore harmony—health—to anyone who is out of tune with the Tao and has thereby incurred illness. But such certainty about acupuncture's salubrious effects is rare in the West, where the method gets mixed reviews. The World Health

Organization lists some forty disorders appropriate for acupuncture, including bronchitis, colitis, diarrhea, and gastritis. But within the West's medical mainstream, opinions about the treatment's efficacy range from the belief that acupuncture is a virtual cure-all, just as its ancient practitioners claimed, to the contention that it is nothing more than outright quackery. Between the two extremes, many Westerners believe that acupuncture works if used in conjunction with an overall lifestyle consistent with good physical and mental health; or that it sometimes works because of its persuasive or hypnotic hold on patients who believe it works; or that it works, but for reasons that its ancient Chinese progenitors could neither have imagined nor understood.

Most American physicians who have experimented with acupuncture have used

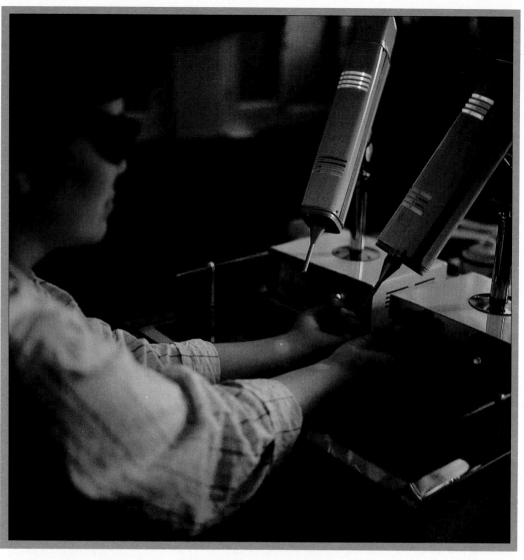

it principally to relieve pain from toothaches, migraine headaches, and neuralgia, and pain caused by bone, muscle, and joint conditions, such as arthritis. Some have used it for cosmetic purposes, maintaining that it can produce some of the same benefits as face-lifts. Still others have tried it in programs for curing nicotine addiction, obesity, insomnia, depression, and even schizophrenia. A New York City doctor whose medical group uses acupuncture along with standard treatments maintains that for pain, acupuncture is "probably the safest treatment, with the fewest side effects and the greatest benefit. It should be the first line of defense, not the last."

Some Western doctors concur about acupuncture's efficacy in easing pain, but they posit reasons far removed from metaphysical rhapsodizing about universal energies and cosmic harmony. In the late 1970s, Western scientists discovered that the brain produces certain chemicals, among them enkephalins and endorphins, that act somewhat like morphine; they are the body's natural painkillers and tranquilizers. Cambridge professor Joseph Needham, an English biochemist and physiologist whom the *New York Review of Books* called "the world's preeminent authority on Chinese science," speculated that acupuncture stimulates the nervous system in ways that step up the release of these naturally occurring analgesics. If this theory—now embraced by a number of other researchers throughout the world—is correct, it bolsters the case that acupuncture, even stripped of its philosophical trappings, is a potent weapon for controlling pain. The theory would also explain why the technique seems promising as a treatment for drug addicts: It would, in effect, stimulate the replacement of natural opiates lost when certain drugs, such as heroin, are introduced into the body.

Dr. E. Gray Dimond is among several Western doctors who have witnessed just how potent a painkiller acupuncture can be. Dimond was chairman of the Health Sciences Department at the University of Missouri Medical School in 1971 when he visited China and observed ten surgical operations in which acupuncture was the only anesthetic used. In one instance, a man had half of a lung removed while sedated by means of a single steel needle inserted and twirled at an acupoint on his left arm. Dimond reported that "the patient's chest was wide open. I could see his heart beating, and all this time the man continued to talk to us cheerfully with total coherence. Halfway through the operation he said he was hungry so the doctors stopped working and gave him a can of fruit to eat."

Despite such reports, many Western physicians still attribute acupuncture's apparent analgesic qualities to some mind-over-matter phenomenon. Either it is a form of hypnotism, they say, or it is a placebo—the Eastern equivalent of the sugar pill. Of course, in the case of any sort of a placebo, the belief itself sometimes produces discernible benefits, if not actual cures. Professor Needham called attention to a fairly recent discovery that the placebo effect itself may play some part in activating the release of endorphins and other palliative brain chemicals.

The problem with all the arguments that seek to dismiss acupuncture by challenging its metaphysical or philosophical validity is this: By positing other ways in which it *might* work, Western critics are necessarily conceding that it *does* work, to whatever extent and for whatever reason. There are, however, experts who simply contend that it does not work at all. One outspoken critic is Petr Skrabanek, Ph.D., of Mater Misericordiae Hospital in Dublin, who bases his attack on the fact that there has been virtually no conceptual development in the theory of acupuncture in thousands of years. "Its antiquity is also its undoing," he says, suggesting a comparison between the dynamic tradition of Western medicine, in which theories and practices are constantly changing as experiments reveal new discoveries, and the static Eastern approach, which relies on time-tested philosophical concepts that are regarded as absolute truths.

Skrabanek also complains about the lack of objective evaluation of acupuncture. Its adherents, he says, manifest a will to believe in the oriental mystique that far outstrips their willingness to pause and think. The Chinese government's figures of 99 percent success of acupuncture in various disorders, he says, "are fictional and on a par with election results in totalitarian countries." His observation agrees with that of many Western scientists who argue that, by occidental standards, there is no known repeatable, empirical proof of the legitimacy of acupuncture or of most other alternative healing methods practiced in the East.

Nevertheless, there are some arguments to counter such criticisms of acupuncture. Skeptics who contend the technique's worth rests with hypnotism or some other manifestation of the power of suggestion, for instance, might have difficulty explaining the growing popularity of the method in the treatment of animals, which are hardly susceptible to suggestion. The acupuncturist at the Wild Bird Care Center in Fort Lauderdale, Florida, asserts that treating creatures who can have no expectations of a cure has "proved to me that acupuncture has physiological effects

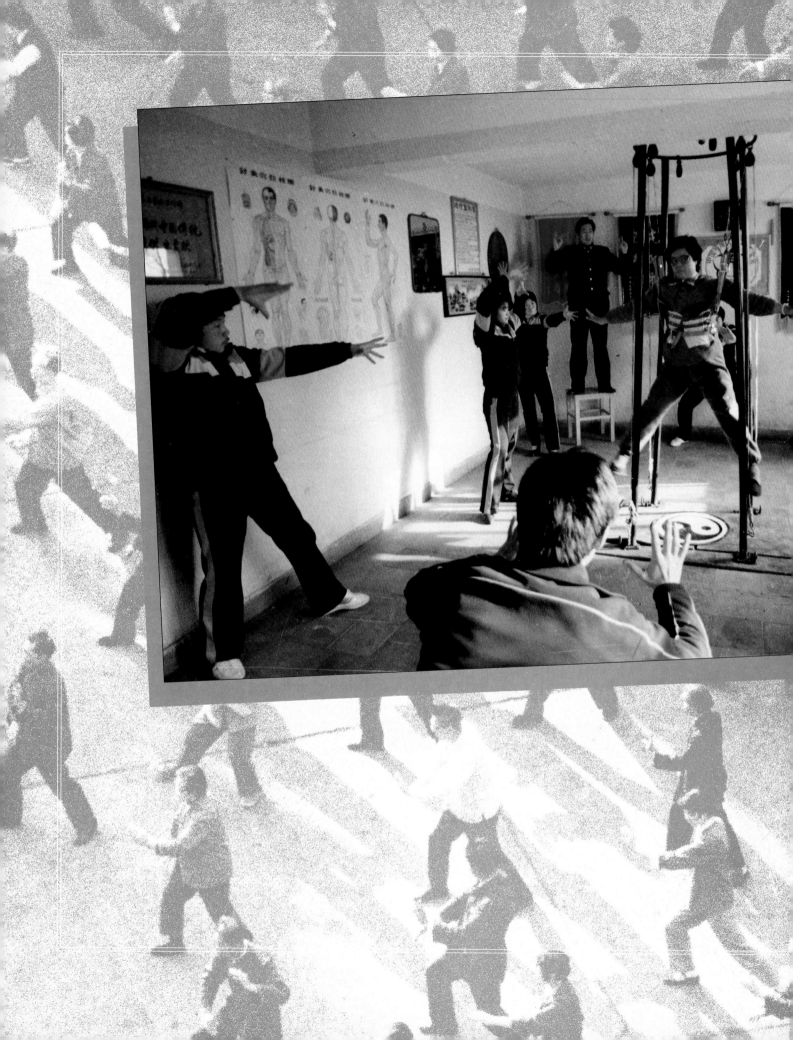

The Quiet Power of Qigong

According to legend, the sixth-century-BC Chinese philosopher and founder of Taoism, Laozi (or Lao-tzu), began each day by visualizing his qi as it traveled through his body's meridians. Laozi became so attuned to this subtle ebb and flow that he could detect any disease-causing imbalance in the qi and repair it by conscious manipulation. Many believe this practice was responsible for his longevity: He supposedly lived for over 100 years.

Laozi's method of sensing and controlling qi is known as *qigong*—"to work the qi." Qigong consists of patterned breathing and stylized physical movements performed while visualizing the energy flow. Some describe the qi as a pressure or a liquid fire coursing through the body. Those who claim full control over the vital flow are qigong masters: Like Laozi, they allegedly move their qi at will, even channeling its force out of the body.

Qigong exercises usually take two forms: Chinese martial arts, where powerful qi energy and physical strength are joined for combat; and healing, where qi is used to restore oneself and others. A qigong master can reportedly transmit restorative qi through his or her hands to people whose depleted stores of qi have left them either weak or ill.

Qigong was banned in China during the Cultural Revolution of the 1960s but now is enjoying a renaissance, with an enthusiastic following of some 60 million people. It is also attracting attention from abroad. Foreigners are lining up in China for training courses and demonstrations in qigong's therapeutic benefits. A medical conference on qigong, held in Beijing in October 1988, was attended by 600 researchers from around the world. Investors are expressing interest in the ancient art as well, with one United States company underwriting a Sino-American qigong rehabilitation center.

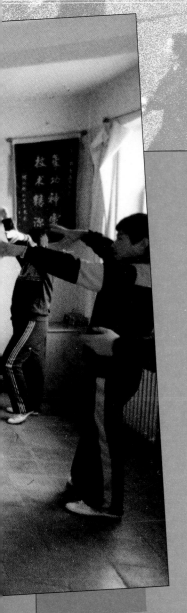

Qigong trainees at a Beijing medical clinic (above) direct their healing qi to the shattered kneecap of a patient suspended over the yin-yang symbol. Critics worry that qigong's growing popularity will slow modernization of the health system in China.

At dawn, a dedicated group (background picture) performs t'ai chi along Shanghai's waterfront. A marriage of qigong theory and slow martial-arts movements, t'ai chi is thought to revitalize every body cell.

A qigong therapist in Beijing (right) imparts his healing energy to a seventy-year-old victim of lung cancer. Chinese cancer patients report improvement in appetite and reduction in levels of pain as a result of the daily qigong treatments they receive.

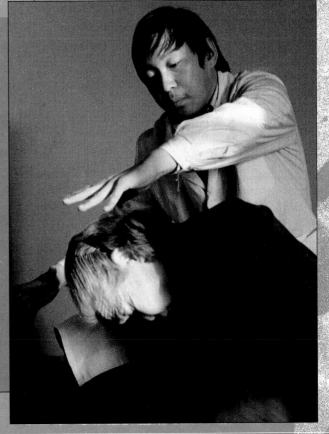

on the body." Some veterinarians, like some physicians, use acupuncture to alleviate pain. A veterinarian in San Diego, for example, uses the Eastern method in treating arthritis. He prefers the needle technique to administering the hormone cortisone, whose negative side effects can include bone loss, hair loss, and muscle softening. In specific rebuttal to the theory that acupuncture used on humans is a form of hypnotism, its defenders argue that hypnotized patients usually seem drowsy and lethargic, while acupuncture patients generally remain alert and clear minded.

As to acupuncture's lack of an empirical foundation, its supporters point out that the therapy does boast a large and highly detailed library of clinical observations, compiled over thousands of years, summarizing what does and does not work. Although this does not amount to empirical evidence in Western terms, the argument can be made that it does constitute statistical validation.

Even the mystical notion of a meridian system has some proponents in the West. One of them is Dr. Robert D. Becker, an American physician and medical writer who has done pioneering research on the relationship between electrical currents and the regeneration of tissue. Becker theorizes that health is maintained by a balanced flow of electromagnetic energy through the body. His experiments, he reports, show that half the acupoints demonstrate relatively high electroconductivity, acting as tiny amplifiers of the electromagnetic energy flowing into the central nervous system. Becker declared he was "sufficiently impressed" by the findings "to conclude that the major aspects of the acupuncture-energetic system" are "objectively verifiable."

Experts with a conciliatory view sometimes point out that cultural and semantic differences tend to overshadow basic commonalities in Western and Eastern healing. Obviously, it is hard for a literal-minded Western doctor accustomed to Greek and Latin terminology to deal with such Chinese diagnoses as "internal fire, weak blood" or "internal wind, excessive phlegm." Still, argue the conciliators, the two traditions may not be so very far apart. Professor

Barry Kahan, physician, Ph.D., and faculty member at the University of Texas Medical School in Houston, has observed that yin-yang has many analogues in Western medicine. He cites the intricate regulation and control mechanisms of the immune system, in which suppressors (yin) and helper (yang) T cells, or lymphocytes, are in opposition, yet are totally interdependent. An imbalance of either cell population can result in disease. "For me, the most interesting aspect of yin and yang is the concept of unity, because there is a unity within the immune response, with many modulations and fine tunings," Kahan says.

American physician Yasuo Ishida, an obstetrician and gynecologist at St. Mary's Health Center, St. Louis, has observed that in the absence of high technology, it is amazing how much the Chinese knew about diseases 2,000 years ago. But their practice of rooting all knowledge in yin-yang metaphysics, Ishida says, has hobbled Chinese healing in its search for acceptance in the West. Ishida himself does not accept many of acupuncture's more extravagant claims to cure conditions ranging from diarrhea to infertility. Nevertheless, he feels that in managing pain, especially in such dire situations as crippling arthritis or terminal cancer, the "quality of life can be better maintained with acupuncture/ moxibustion than by having the central nervous system knocked out with narcotics, or having gastrointestinal bleeding as a side effect of some potent antiarthritic drugs."

Whatever its faults or virtues, Eastern healing's popularity is growing in the West. Some doctors are being besieged with requests for acupuncture, and in an increasing number of clinics, Western techniques exist side by side with Chinese or Indian methods.

In trendy California, acupuncture's popularity has been augmented in recent decades by an enthusiastic celebrity following. Actress Jaclyn Smith, for example, credited one Hollywood acupuncturist, Zion Yu, with ridding her of neck pain that resulted from a traffic accident. Other Hollywood notables enthusiastic about Yu included actress Jane Fonda, actors James Garner and Robert Wagner, and ex-Beatle George Harrison. For all his popularity, however,

Shiatsu: A Healing Pressure on the Acupoints

In an attempt to modernize Japanese medicine during the American occupation after World War II, General Douglas MacArthur banned traditional oriental medical practices, including a form of massage called shiatsu. The defeated population had submitted to most American dictates, but this went too far. The Japanese association for the blind asked Helen Keller to intervene on behalf of the many blind shiatsu masseurs left unemployed. Her efforts led President Truman to pressure MacArthur into revoking the ban.

Modern shiatsu experts see this as an example of the continuing conflict between Eastern and Western medicine. Most Westerners are reluctant to classify massage as a necessary medical treatment rather than a luxury. But shiatsu, the most common form of Eastern massage, differs in theory and application from its Western counterparts: While a Swedish massage uses a vigorous rubdown to ease muscle tension, shiatsu consists of concentrated, static pressure on localized points to heal body and soul.

In fact, shiatsu is considered a complement to other oriental forms of healing, such as acupuncture and moxibustion. These treatments all purportedly regulate the flow of animating energy responsible for health. And all three treat identical points along the unseen energy pathways, or meridians, traversing the body.

The term *shiatsu* translates literally as "finger pressure," but most practitioners also use their elbows or feet to bear down on the energy points, called *tsubos* in Japan. Some will also stretch or rotate a patient's limbs during treatment. Although this healing method can be painful, followers swear by the results, visiting shiatsu therapists for a wide variety of disorders, which range from migraines, insomnia, and diarrhea to muscle fatigue and backache.

A reflexology therapist's hands (above) palpate a patient's foot. Reflexology—a type of shiatsu that focuses on feet and hands—holds that tenderness in an extremity signals blocked energy, believed to cause illness.

New York shiatsu instructor Wataru Ohashi, here ministering to ballet dancer Ivan Nagy, first diagnoses an ailment as possessing either yin or yang qualities; then he applies pressure to the body's energy points, or tsubos. When treating a yang disorder, Ohashi's pressure opposes the subtle energy currents; if the problem is yin in character, he works with the energy flow.

A Chinese physician evaluates a patient's pulses in this early-nineteenth-century watercolor. Each of the twelve distinct pulses recognized by Chinese medicine—six per wrist—is linked with a vital organ. Terms such as slippery, tight, and tardy-irregular describe a pulse and give clues to its organ's condition.

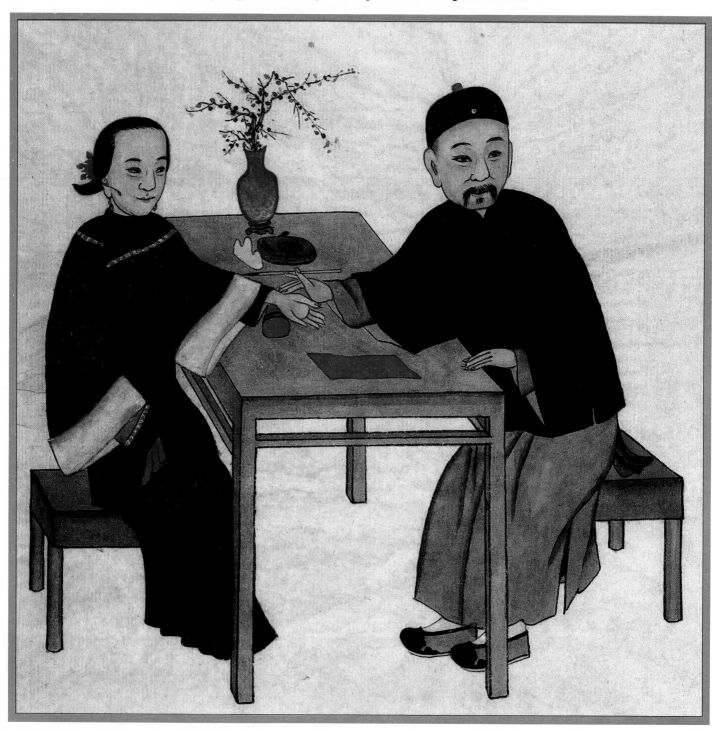

Yu was not without critics in the medical establishment, who contended he was practicing medicine without a license. In 1975, the Taipei-bred acupuncturist found a powerful ally, however, in then-Governor Jerry Brown, who saw to it that California explicitly legalized Yu's practice. In the following decade, in most large cities in California and elsewhere, acupuncturists were no longer a rarity, and people of diverse backgrounds sought them out to augment—or even replace—more orthodox medical practitioners.

One proposed explanation for the upsurge in the acceptance of acupuncture and other Eastern treatments is that, despite its incredible advances, Western medicine does not satisfy everyone. Its critics cite the cool impersonality of the purely scientific approach, along with spiraling costs, drugs that sometimes lead to dependency or have unforeseen and even catastrophic side effects, and an excessive reliance on quick-fix surgery with the concomitant neglect of gentler treatment that might prove equally effective. Moreover, faith-based healing can be especially appealing in the promise it holds for sufferers of diseases as yet untreatable or incurable by Western medicine.

Another possible factor in the newfound popularity of Eastern therapies might be their inclusion in the panoply of neo-mystical enthusiasms that come under the umbrella of the New Age. Holistic medicine is a New Age mainstay, as is the tendency to reject scientific orthodoxy in favor of exotic alternative therapies—especially if those therapies feature metaphysical connections, as the Eastern techniques do. Regrettably, the increasing willingness of many to seek alternative healing has brought with it unscrupulous practitioners with no real knowledge of medical techniques, Eastern or Western.

Be it panacea or quackery or something in between those extremes, acupuncture does not stand by itself in the Chinese medicinal scheme of things. It is but one tool, often used in conjunction with several others, to keep the mind, body, and spirit properly attuned. And, in classical practice, none of the tools is used until the patient has undergone an elaborate—and distinctly Eastern—process of diagnosis.

Since the main thrust of all Chinese healing is preventive rather than curative, diagnosis of an impending dysfunction ideally comes before major symptoms of disease manifest themselves. It is said that a skilled healer can pick up clues from such subtle indicators as a patient's walking gait, a discordant quality in the voice or breathing, emotional or dietary changes, or certain nervous habits. If potential problems are spotted from such minute hints, the reasoning goes, impending illness can be averted. If matters are further along, however, a more formal diagnosis is in order.

Refined over the centuries, the diagnosis consists of the "four examinations": inspecting, asking questions, touching, and listening and smelling. (Smelling, by which practitioners were once said to glean considerable information from odors of the body and breath, is less used today; more varied diets, which affect odors, have confused the issue, as have changing hygiene and perfumes and cosmetics that mask natural odors.) As part of the inspection phase, the physician pays particular attention to examining the tongue. The thickness, coloration, and coating of the tongue are said to provide data on the state of the circulatory and digestive systems. The intensive questioning phase elicits information about the patient's symptoms.

The most important step in the examination comes under the heading of touching and involves taking the pulse—the pulses, in fact, since classical Chinese healing distinguishes not one pulse, as Western medicine does, but a total of twelve. There are six in each wrist, three on the surface and three deeper at specific points along the radial artery. In the classical Chinese tradition, the twelve pulses correspond to the twelve internal organs. In the West, the pulse yields information primarily about the state of the patient's cardiovascular system. But to a doctor of Chinese medicine, the pulses purport to provide a complete picture of an individual's physical health. And it is said that a skilled practitioner can also read in the pulses past and future illnesses. Along with the incredible range of information they supposedly yield, the pulses are also said to be the final arbiter in formulating a diagnosis. The classic treatise on internal Chinese medicine, and probably the oldest medical book in existence, is the *Nei Ching,* also called the *Yellow Emperor's Classic of Internal Medicine.* It is thought to have been composed during the reign of Huang Ti, the Yellow Emperor, probably between the years 2697 BC and 2597 BC. "Nothing surpasses the examination of the pulse," that tome relates, "for with it errors cannot be committed."

Touching also involves palpation of the patient's abdomen and of places called "alarm points," usually at sites over vital organs, to pick up additional clues about systemic functioning. The listening aspect of the diagnostic procedure concerns itself primarily with the patient's spiritual and mental states and how they bear on his or her physical health. Tone of voice and ways of phrasing are two factors the practitioner looks for in assessing the patient's personality and habits of thought.

On the basis of the four examinations, the physician preliminarily groups the patient's symptoms into what are called the eight principal patterns. These are yin and yang, along with three more sets of interacting opposites that partake of yin or yang: interior and exterior, deficiency and excess, and cold and hot. These, in turn, are divided into various subcategories before a clinical syndrome is defined.

Chinese medicine traditionally describes disorders in terms of the five elements, or energy phases. Wood, a metaphor for generation, growth, and renewal, is the category for ailments of the liver. Fire, the element of warmth, transformation, and change, governs the blood, heart, and mind. Earth, the source of food, corresponds to the digestive system and spleen. Metal, particularly gold, expressing the bodily "shine" that results from proper oxygenation, is the category for the lungs. And water, the nourisher of life, corresponds to the generative organs.

Once the patient is diagnosed, the healer prescribes treatment. Either acupuncture or moxibustion is likely to figure in the cure, usually in conjunction with other therapies. In fact, the *Nei Ching* lays out four approaches to treatment besides acupuncture or moxibustion: Heal the spirit; nourish the body; unite the whole body, mind, and spirit; and give medication. Physiotherapy or breathing exercises may be prescribed for various ailments of the body, along with meditation to help correct problems of the spirit. It is even more probable that the practitioner will turn to two other bastions of Chinese healing, herbal medicine and special diet. With herbal healing, as with acupuncture, the healer must have considerable knowledge and an expert touch, for Chinese herbal practice is amazingly complex.

Calculating exactly how many plants the Chinese use in healing is difficult. Five thousand is a reasonable estimate, and these may have subdivisions: Some are used whole and some divided into component parts—roots, stems, seeds, flowers, or leaves. Each part may be used for a different purpose. Locally grown vegetation is deemed to be the most efficacious, and many of the healing plants are grown throughout China's vast southern provinces. Some are cultivated, but it is said that the best ones grow wild. Their harvesting and processing has changed little in more than 3,000 years. They must be located, gathered, sorted, washed, separated into component parts, dried, and stored. Modern technology's contribution allows for extracting and refining useful ingredients to increase potency. In the classical style, however, the plants are brewed into tonics or potions that can be taken orally. Some modern variations allow for injection, but these are not common.

Chinese healers believe certain herbs have affinities for certain organs, but that notion is only the starting point for herbal medicine's intricacies. In the West, the assumption is that a medicine shown to prevent or cure disease in one person will probably have the same effect in another. But there is no such standardization in the Eastern tradition, in which some 16,000 possible herbal prescriptions must be tailored specifically for each individual. An American physician who has traveled to China for extensive study of Chinese traditional medicine, Dr. David Eisenberg of Harvard Medical School, notes that if a case of pneumonia re-

The Root That Is Said to Cure Everything

The most widely used medicinal herb in Asia, if not in the world, is ginseng. The seemingly limitless benefits of this gnarled root were first recorded in about 2800 BC, in one of the earliest Chinese herbal catalogs; since then ginseng has been used to treat almost every affliction known to humanity. In fact, while its name in Chinese means "man plant," because its roots often resemble a human form, ginseng's botanical name, *Panax pseudoginseng,* translates as "remedy for all."

The versatile root can be steeped into a faintly bitter tea, ground into a powder, or chewed as is. However administered, ginseng supposedly treats a host of unrelated ailments, including diabetes, asthma, anemia, and hyperten-sion. It is also consumed as an aphrodisiac, as well as a stress reducer and an aging retardant. In fact, ginseng proponents claim it is unique in its ability to adapt to the body's needs. Thus it is used as a pick-me-up during the day and a sleep inducer at night.

Scientific analysis of this adaptable plant has been complicated by its complex chemical structure. The root does contain pharmacologically active ingredients that might account for some of its purported effects. However, scientists remain unconvinced of the efficacy of ginseng. And some cite cases of ginseng abuse, with patients suffering depression, confusion, or insomnia from an overdose of the plant.

Ginseng may still be a mystery to Western scientists, but it is a familiar one; the root has been known to Westerners for centuries. It is indigenous to the eastern United States and Canada and has been traded with the Far East since the 1700s. George Washington mentioned it in his diary: "Passing over the [Appalachian] Mountains, I met a number of Persons and Pack horses going in with Ginseng." Today American farmers purvey over 200,000 pounds to Asia each year.

The roots are priced according to various factors, including variety, age, color, and shape—a human contour is deemed most valuable. American ginseng generally fetches between $80 to $100 a pound, making annual exports of it worth almost $20 million. But a pound of wild Korean ginseng can sell for over $300. And roots with a particularly exotic form, such as the one pictured here, have commanded a market price of up to $10,000 an ounce.

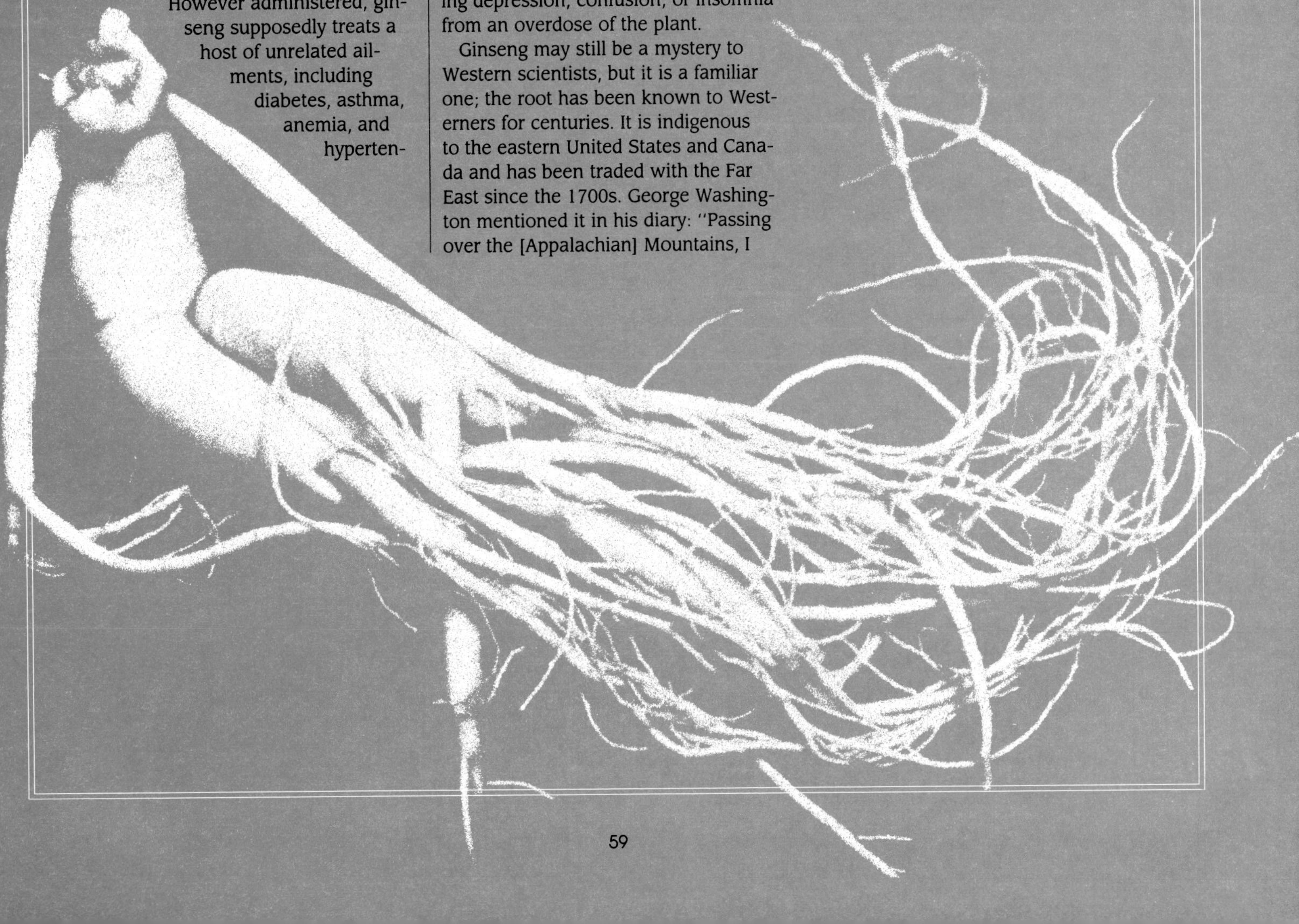

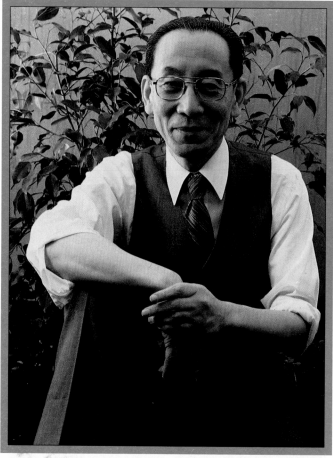

sponds dramatically within hours to a single combination of herbs, the next step for a Western researcher would be to test these same herbs on fifty more pneumonia patients in order to measure the treatment's effectiveness. In China, however, the doctor would prescribe different combinations of herbs for each of the fifty patients.

On the whole, Western medicine has tended to regard much of the Chinese herbal pharmacopoeia as fanciful, with some exceptions for those items having scientifically established value. Certain iodine-bearing seaweeds, for example, are used in China to treat enlargement of the thyroid gland, just as iodine is used to treat thyroid anomalies in the West. The willow plant, which contains salicylic acid—the chemical basis for aspirin—has long been used in the East for rheumatic aches and pains. Mulberry flowers containing rutin help in combating high blood pressure. Proponents estimate that some 90 percent of Chinese remedies may also contain massive doses of vitamins and minerals, giving them valid healing powers independent of their folkloric and mythical origins.

Consistent with the notion that good health exists in an overall matrix of proper living, diet has always been an important component of healing in China and elsewhere in the Orient, a way of incorporating the Tao into everyday life. Chinese dietary theory relies on the conviction that, as mother of all life, the earth is the source of basic nutrition.

Advocates note that for the Western world, a similar idea is contained in the biblical statement that man is made of dust (earth)—a truth substantiated by modern chemistry, insofar as earth means all chemical elements. The Chinese reason that vegetables assimilate inorganic matter and produce organic substances, such as carbohydrates, proteins, or fats, while animals live off these products, breaking them down for their own physiological construction and energy. Meat eating, therefore, is an indirect, or artificial, avenue to nutrition. Even so, the Chinese healing tradition does not require a strictly vegetarian diet. Beef, pork, chicken, and other animal proteins not only are allowed, but also are carefully categorized according to the effects they have on the body once their nutritional elements enter various meridians and organs.

In the Indian medical tradition and in some Japanese schools of thought, however, vegetarianism is held to be necessary to optimum well-being. It is said that when properly selected, cooked, and eaten, vegetables can provide good nutrition and exert certain curative powers. Grains, beans, and vegetables may contain fewer amino acids—the building blocks of protein—than animal products, yet they are considered far superior foods for human beings. As long as people eat animals and animal products, some Indian and Japanese dietary purists say, human sickness will persist, and human beings will never be happy.

Eastern dietary philosophy made itself felt in the West in recent years under Japanese aegis in the form of macrobiotics, a system based on the blending harmonies of yin and yang. In fact, macrobiotics was a major impetus behind the current Western craze for natural foods. Its prime progenitor was George Ohsawa, a Japanese business-school graduate with an abiding interest in philosophy and healing. Ohsawa called his system Zen macrobiotics, after the Buddhist sect. The plan recommended a diet that progressed through ten increasingly restrictive phases until brown rice was the only food eaten. Brown rice, Ohsawa contended, was the food in which yin and yang were most perfectly balanced. Unfortunately, brown rice, however nutritious, proved insufficient by itself to sustain life. A number of the early macrobiotic faithful became malnourished and ill, and some eventually died.

A much less restrictive macrobiotic diet was devised by one of Ohsawa's followers, Michio Kushi, who dropped "Zen" from the name and stressed that good health, physical and spiritual, is for all humankind. (He notes that the term *macrobiotics* comes from the Greek *makrobios*—"great life" or "long life"—the name given to the regimen recommended by Hippocrates, the father of Western medicine.) Kushi followed the notion that foods may be grouped according to their content of yin or yang and used to maintain the proper yin-yang balance of the individual. However, his flexible version of macrobiotics added a range of foods to Ohsawa's brown rice staple. The diet has certain geographical variations, since locally grown foods are regarded as part of the total environment of a person living in a specific region. But for those living in a temperate climate—the prevailing climate for most Western countries—the Kushi diet relies heavily on whole grains, which make up about half the total food intake and are recommended for consumption in some form at every meal. Most of the rest of the diet is made up of legumes, other garden vegetables, and sea vegetables, often consumed in the form of soup. Fruit can be eaten occasionally, and even meat is not completely ruled out. Fish can be eaten two or three times a week, if the macrobiotic dieter so desires. In addition, the sparing use of roasted seeds or nuts is permitted, along with moderate quantities of sesame or corn oil, or any other natural vegetable oil.

Although Kushi did formulate an elaborate food plan, he stressed that macrobiotics is not merely a diet. "Macrobiotics means the universal way of life with which humanity has developed biologically, psychologically, and spiritually and with which we will maintain our health, freedom, and happiness," Kushi has written. "Macrobiotics includes a dietary approach but its purpose is to ensure the survival of the human race and its further evolution on this planet."

Its grand vision notwithstanding, the dietary component of Kushi's macrobiotic life has its critics in both East and West. Chinese medicine recommends a diet much more varied than the macrobiotic regimen, a plan based on five food groups that are thought to nourish five of the "solid" organs. Macrobiotics, in the Chinese view, is not fully nutritional. In the West, experts find Kushi's macrobiotic diet to be admirably low in fat, especially in artery-threatening, low-density cholesterol, and high in beneficial fiber. They find some basis, therefore, in devotees' claim that macrobiotics can be a potent preventive of arterial diseases and heart attacks. Certainly, in that regard macrobiotic fare seems healthier than the average American diet, in which 40 percent of all calories come from fat. Still, Western doctors are skeptical of macrobiotics enthusiasts' claim that their diet can prevent cancer or help cancer patients live longer—the message implicit in one of Kushi's books, *The Cancer Prevention Diet.*

The National Cancer Institute resolutely opposes macrobiotic diets, and the American Cancer Society states that, in addition to lacking proof of their worth as cancer preventives, macrobiotic diets can ultimately lead to scurvy, anemia, and protein starvation. And from a purely nutritional standpoint, a number of Western experts find the diet less than ideal, since it tends to be low in calcium, iron, and vitamins D and B-12.

One expert trying to bridge the East-West dietary

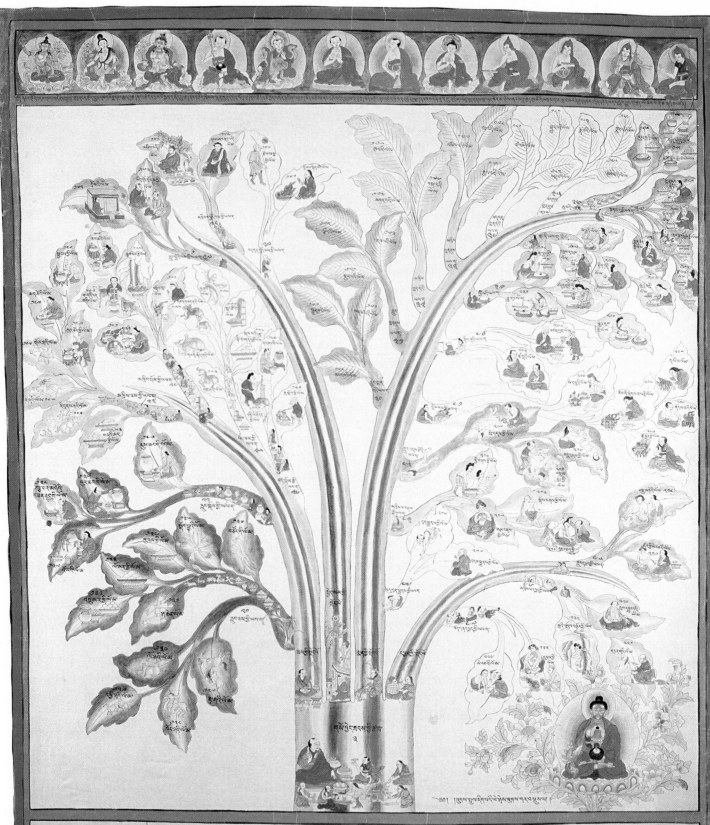

question is Lawrence Kushi, a man who seems to be in an ideal position to make the effort. He is Michio Kushi's son, and he also holds a doctorate in nutrition from the Harvard School of Public Health. Although the younger Kushi upholds what he sees as macrobiotics' virtues, he also concedes that "some definite problems with misconceptions" are involved. "People tend to be evangelical about it," he says. "They think it's the answer to everything. If you eat macrobiotically, nothing bad will happen to you. But nothing's absolute, macrobiotics included."

Young Kushi's observation notwithstanding, much of oriental healing does rest on absolutes. A universe in which yin and yang contend is an absolute that is essential to Asian medicine, for instance. And in Ayurveda, the ancient healing system native to India, an absolute is the dharma, the laws of maintaining oneness with a harmonious cosmic order not so different from the one posited by the Tao. According to both Taoism and Hinduism, the universe is constantly in a state of flux. In the Hindu construct, there is a never-ending cycle of creation, preservation, and destruction—true in nature and, by inference, true in human beings as nature's microcosms. The secret of health is oneness with the natural order—preserving life long and well through proper living, dying when the time comes, being reborn as the cycle wheels anew.

The Sanskrit word for the cosmic order is *veda*. The word is usually translated as "complete knowledge," but the concept is much more inclusive. Veda is the intelligence that underlies all activity in the universe. Like a master blueprint for the cosmic scheme, veda directs all forms and functions—of the universe and everything in it—while remaining itself unchanged and inviolable. Immersed in the natural order of veda, the individual is in accord with the laws of nature and is thus perfectly happy and healthy. This attunement involves one's whole mode of existence and implies thinking, feeling, and acting in positive ways that support life and health.

Like Chinese medicine, Ayurveda—the Sanskrit word

means "knowledge of life" or "science of life"—is old beyond reckoning. In fact, although both disciplines have been codified and transcribed over several millenniums, certain of their elements are rooted in prehistory. As far back as it can be traced, Ayurvedic medicine has its origins in the Vedas, the oldest of Hindu scriptures, and in subsequent sacred commentaries, the Brahmanas, the Aranyakas, and the Upanishads. According to certain Ayurvedic texts, the healing knowledge itself did not derive from the scientific method of observation, hypothesis, and testing but was intuited by sages attuned to the pure cosmic consciousness where all knowledge resides.

A landmark rendering of the Vedic sages' healing lore was made by the famous Indian physician Charaka, a legendary figure who may have lived anytime between the fifth century BC and the first century AD. Thereafter, Ayurveda developed and persisted as the chief among several related healing systems in India until the fifteenth century. Political vicissitudes caused its decline, and some of its important literature was destroyed. But with the coming of Indian independence in the twentieth century, Ayurveda enjoyed a resurgence, which continues today.

During the early days of Indian thought, illness was deemed a punishment inflicted by the gods as retribution for sin. Eventually, however, belief in reincarnation removed the gods as instigators and substituted the idea of karma, the concept that the sum of one's thoughts and actions in one existence determines one's fate in the next. Karma seems to present a paradox for Ayurvedic healers (called *vaidyas*): If health and illness are predestined, what right have doctors to interfere with the course they take? But Ayurveda is notable in that its mystical and magical aspects coexist comfortably with its pragmatic and practical side. The vaidyas conclude that it is their own karmic mission to prevent or alleviate suffering, regardless of its source.

Still, Ayurvedic medicine is both philosophical and holistic in the best oriental tradition. It identifies life as the union of body, sense, mind, and soul, and its ultimate pur-

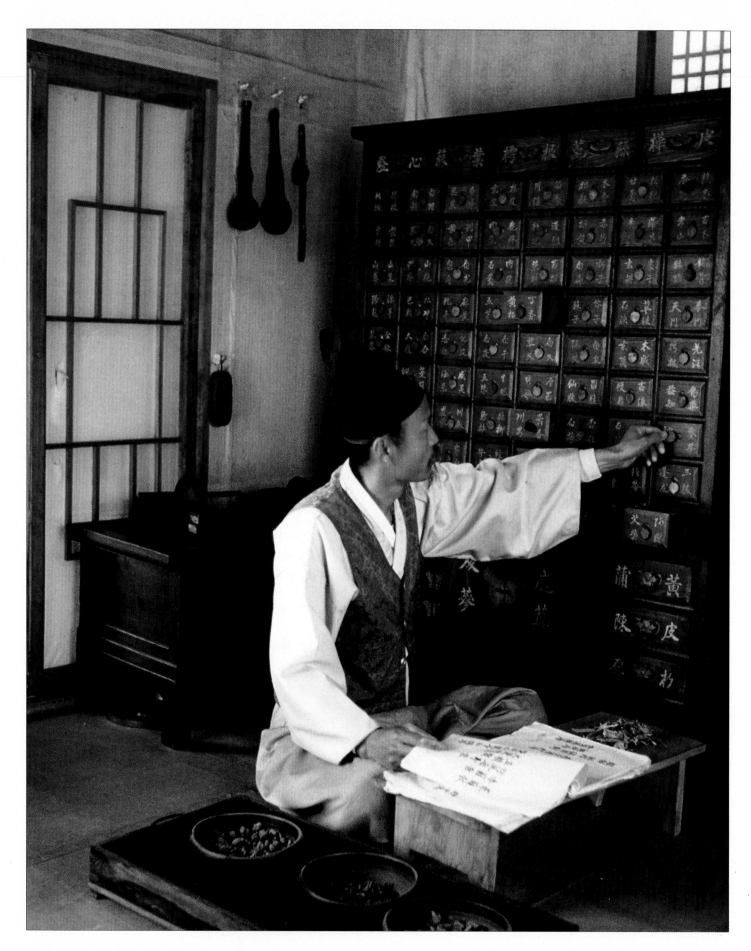

pose reaches beyond physical health to spiritual enlightenment. It describes the proper attunement of the human organism in terms of complex categories and subcategories in which spiritual, mental, physical, and environmental factors coexist and, ideally, harmonize.

In a construct similar to the Chinese concept, Ayurveda holds that the human body is made up of five energy elements, the same five that compose all the universe—earth, water, fire, air, and space. In turn, these five figure in the character of the vital energies that, expressing veda's natural order, animate and regulate the body. These vital energies are called *doshas,* and there are three different types: *vata,* which represents air and lightness and governs the body's motor and nervous functions; *pitta,* the vehicle for metabolism, energy production, and digestion; and *kapha,* which represents earth and water and is a liquid and passive energy that regulates the body's structural element, cohesiveness, and strength. Just as qi flows through meridians in Chinese lore, Ayurveda's doshas operate in the body through subtle channels called *srotas—* "subtle" in the sense that they may be as small as the space between atoms, molecules, and cells. There are also gross srotas, such as the windpipe and digestive tract, which carry nutrients and wastes. As messengers for the five elements, doshas connect each element to one of the five senses. The doshas also govern the metabolic processes producing the "seven bodily constituents": plasma, blood, muscle, fat, bone, marrow,

and in adults, semen or ova.

The proper flow and balance of the doshas is crucial to health in Ayurveda, just as the harmonious flow of qi is essential to well-being in Chinese medicine. And practitioners of Ayurveda, like Chinese physicians, use both diet and herbal medicine as preventives and cures—in the case of the Indian tradition, to assure that vata, pitta, and kapha are kept in balance.

Food is particularly important. One legend has it that a student once asked Charaka if it were true that "diet is half of Ayurveda." "No, that is wrong," the great physician is supposed to have said, "it is almost all of Ayurveda." Foods are categorized based on their apportionment of a certain dosha. Bitter and astringent tastes manifest the presence of vata; while hot, spicy, and pungent are associated with pitta; and sweet, sour, and salty with the energy of kapha. An overabundance or lack of food rich in any one type of energy can disrupt its associated dosha and cause illness. Treatment then takes the form of altering the diet to restore equilibrium. In Ayurvedic reasoning, for example, an excess of hot, spicy pitta foods can cause this dosha to inflame the skin and stomach lining. Balancing relief is available in the form of mangoes or ice cream, representing the pitta-balancing qualities of coolness and sweetness. In devising a diet to maintain good health in a patient, an Ayurvedic healer considers not only the doshic qualities of the food, but those of the patient. People are classified according to ten body types that supposedly express a preponderance of one or more doshas. For instance, one might be a vata type, a vata-

These bamboo medicine sticks allegedly foretold a patient's fate in turn-of-the-century China. A priest, given a numbered stick randomly selected by a sufferer, used it to divine a prognosis that ranged from recovery to death.

pitta type, a kapha-pitta type, and so on. People who have all three in nearly equal measure are vata-pitta-kapha types—"tridoshic" as opposed to "bidoshic" (two types) or "monodoshic" (only one type). Each dosha implies a set of characteristics. Vata types, for example, are said to have light builds and to be vivacious and quick in movement, action, and speech, while pitta people have medium builds, operate at a moderate pace, speak well, but tend to be irritable and angry. Stolid kapha types are said to have heavier builds, great strength and endurance, methodical ways, and tranquil temperaments. Each doshic type is supposed to be prone to particular disorders. Vata people, for example, are said to be particularly susceptible to anxiety, dry skin, insomnia, and hypertension, among other problems. To prevent these conditions, the person is supposed to eat foods that help balance, or "pacify," vata—foods opposite in quality to the characteristics of vata dosha. If a person is bidoshic or tridoshic, there will be a mixture of doshic characteristics and tendencies, and a more intricate balancing required in diet. Body types figure in curative as well as preventive healing, not only in relation to food, but to other Ayurvedic therapies.

Psychology is not neglected in Ayurvedic healing; in fact, the study of the mind is one of its oldest disciplines. Charaka constructed a motivational scheme of life that reduced all human actions to three fundamental drives or goals: longevity and health, the urge for wealth and power, and the attainment of spiritual development. Along with a number of recommended disciplines for mental hygiene, Ayurveda also has dietary treatment for mental problems. Chronic depression, for instance, is thought to result from unbalanced kaphic energy and to require such foods as salad, bone soups, drinks spiced with cloves and ginger, and items that are rich in honey and cinnamon—all of them filled with rectifying vata or pitta.

Like diet, herbal medicine follows the dictates of the doshas. Medicinal plants are classified according to taste, as well as to their qualities of hot and cold—attributes related not to temperature, but to corresponding doshic potencies. Vata and kapha are cold, pitta is hot. Herbal prescriptions—and they are virtually innumerable—aim at galvanizing one of the three energies by supplementing it with a corresponding potency or by subduing it with an opposing potency. For example, ginger—a hot potency—is thought to be effective against colds and flu—ailments showing an excess of cold vata or kapha.

Along with calculations for taste and for hot and cold potencies, vaidyas prescribing diet and medicine must contend with another wrinkle—the ability of the taste qualities to change during the process of digestion. A food that tastes like kapha (sweet) or pitta (sour) in the mouth might change to vata (bitter) somewhere during its alimentary journey. And, as if the equation were not by now sufficiently complex, there is also a matter of seasonal variations. Doshas' potencies are thought to rise and fall in seasonal curves. Light, dry, cold, and mobile vata reaches its maximum activity in the fall; dry, hot, oily pitta peaks in summer; and cold, heavy, liquid kapha increases in winter. Moreover, the doshas can become unbalanced not only by external factors such as climate and diet, but by internal causes such as karma-dimming improper thoughts and actions. Thoughts can change the quality of food. Thus cleanliness and purity of mind and body are basic to the Ayurvedic concept of health, which entails a variety of purification rituals for mental and physical well-being. Those aimed at protecting the physical body involve elimination, purging, vomiting, and techniques of internal cleansing. These practices aim mainly at keeping the gross srotas unblocked.

The most basic Ayurvedic technique for mental hygiene is meditation, whose purpose is to allow the mind to experience a silent, expanded state beyond thought—the state of consciousness that is the substratum of veda and the source of mind.

Ayurveda has no construct that corresponds exactly to the Chinese notion of acupoints through which the body's animating energy can be manipulated. However, Indian tradition does posit the existence of *marmas*, particular points

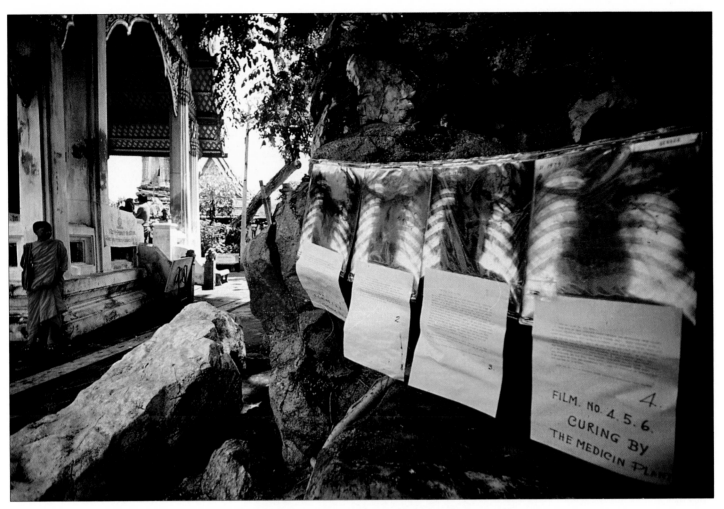

*Outside a temple at Wat Po, Bangkok's center for folk healing,
x-rays hanging from a banyan tree publicize the progress of a patient suffering
from tuberculosis. With the aid of such modern diagnostic tools,
healers formulate a course of treatment consisting
entirely of traditional folk cures, such as the drawing of magical diagrams,
or the administration of pills made from pulverized sacred writings.*

on the body where injury proves lethal or does serious damage. The marma theory has not held up very well under scientific scrutiny; some of these points do indeed lie over vital organs, nerves, or blood vessels, but others do not. Still, some modern students of Ayurveda are returning to ancient texts for deeper study of the 108 marmas. One school of thought holds that the marmas are points where the link between mind and body, and perhaps between the body and the universal order, is particularly vital. The theory goes that removing blockages at the marmas might enhance health and even cure disease.

All the fluctuation and interplay inherent in Ayurveda reflect the basic Hindu concept of a fluctuating and interdependent universe. They also make the practice of this ancient form of healing a challenging art. Its diagnostic tools are characteristically complicated. A cursory examination entails eight steps. The initial one is taking the pulse, which

even in the most superficial reading is said to provide a plethora of information about the state of the doshas. A light and rapid beat shows disruption of the vata, while a disturbed pitta registers in a jumpy pulse, and an afflicted kapha in a slow, heavy beat. Subsequent phases of the examination involve checking the eyes, the temperature of the ears, the texture and color of the tongue and the skin, the color of the mouth, the voice's pitch and volume, as well as the patient's urine. As in Chinese medicine, almost every characteristic of the patient's appearance, mental and emotional attitudes, and behavior is held to be a clue to his or her state of health.

Ayurveda has been slow in making its way to the West, partly because it only revived slowly in its own country and efforts to integrate its ways with the Western scientific tradition have been comparatively slow. (China was quicker to unite its classical methods with occidental ways;

A traditional Ayurvedic doctor, or vaidya, dispenses herbal medications in a contemporary Indian clinic. Ayurveda dominates the country's health-care system, claiming 70 percent of the population as patients. They are essentially a captive audience, however, for in the rural areas of India, Ayurveda is the only medicine practiced.

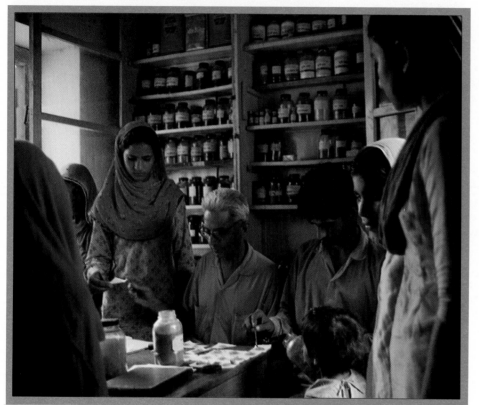

often both disciplines are practiced in the same hospital or clinic.) In India today, however, an effort is under way to retrieve and test the ancient lore. There are nearly 500,000 Ayurvedic practitioners in India, and Ayurveda is taught along with Western medicine in Indian universities. In addition, efforts are in progress to subject Ayurvedic herbal remedies to clinical testing—a lengthy procedure because some 8,000 formulas are involved. (There is a story that an ancient Ayurvedic sage tested his students by having them seek out plants that could not be used medicinally. One pupil returned empty-handed, saying he could not find such a plant. This student passed the test.) The World Health Organization is supporting worldwide development of Ayurveda on the premise that its inexpensive methods might prove beneficial in less affluent nations. And, in recent years, Ayurvedic clinics have begun to spring up in America.

Ayurveda's reception from the West's traditional med-

ical community has been cautious and skeptical. The chief complaint, as with Chinese healing, is that there is little or no scientific basis or support for it. Even so, some highly reputable doctors in the United States, Europe, and South America have begun to take an interest in the Ayurvedic arts. One such physician is Nancy Lonsdorf, medical director of the Maharishi Ayurveda Medical Center in Washington, D.C., a clinic that offers both Ayurvedic and Western treatment. Dr. Lonsdorf received her medical degree from Johns Hopkins Medical School and took postgraduate training in psychiatry at Stanford University. Although she has in no way abandoned her occidental training, Lonsdorf feels that Ayurveda's holistic approach provides a dimension that Western medicine lacks. Also enthusiastic is Dr. John Canary, professor of medicine and director of endocrine research at Georgetown University Medical School in Washington, D.C. Canary combines his career in Western medicine with the study of Ayurveda and of traditional healing methods in various other cultures. "Many aspects of traditional medicine," he contends, "should have a place in our medical armamentarium," alongside computer technology, hormone therapy, and radiation treatment.

If Ayurveda is still a comparative stranger to the West, Yoga is a familiar acquaintance. This ancient practice—reflected in both the Hinduism and Buddhism that are practiced in India, and thought by some to be older than both—became a subculture staple during the blossoming neo-mysticism in the United States and parts of Europe in the 1960s. Some of its many variations remain highly popular among modern New Age enthusiasts.

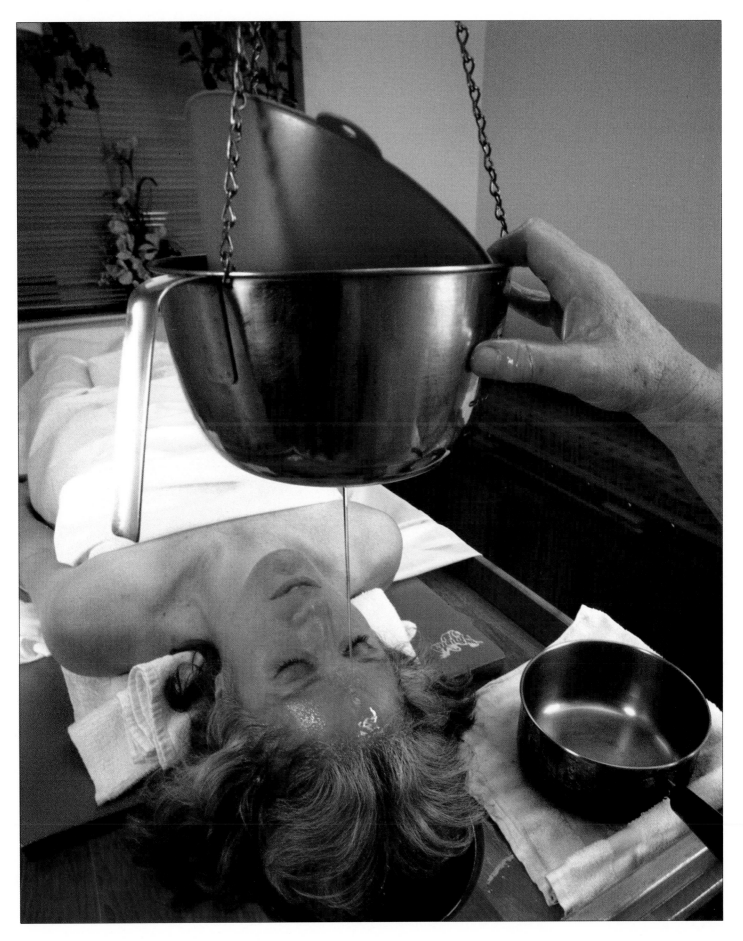

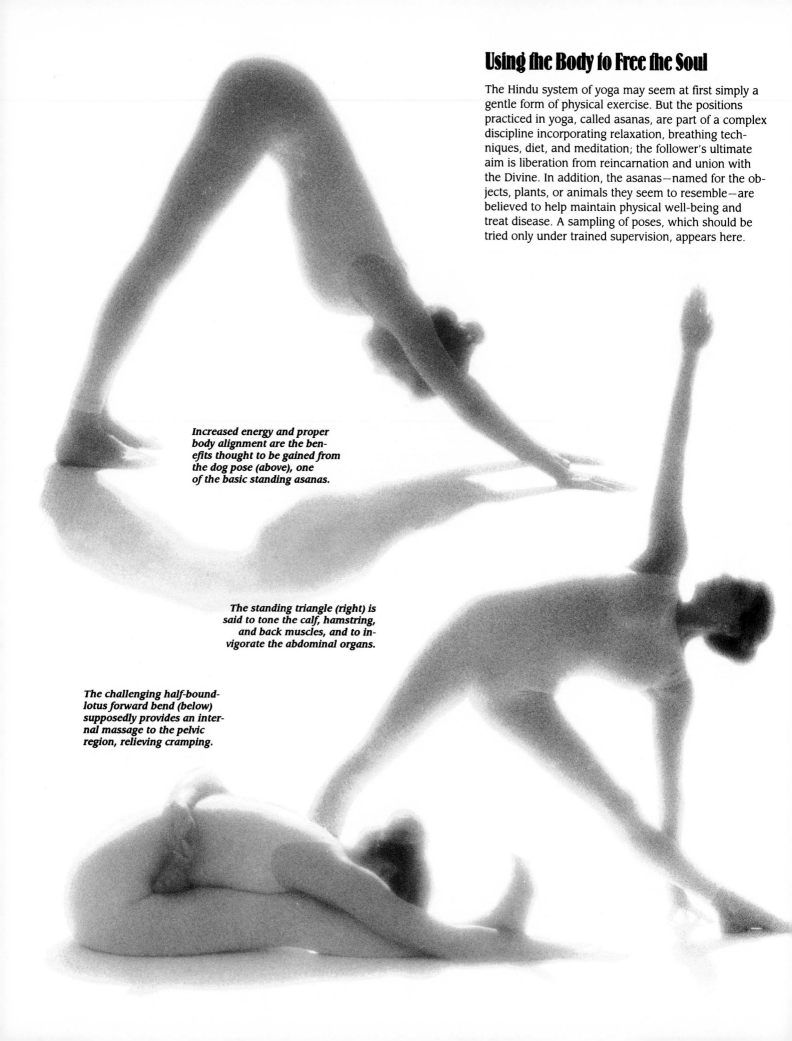

Using the Body to Free the Soul

The Hindu system of yoga may seem at first simply a gentle form of physical exercise. But the positions practiced in yoga, called asanas, are part of a complex discipline incorporating relaxation, breathing techniques, diet, and meditation; the follower's ultimate aim is liberation from reincarnation and union with the Divine. In addition, the asanas—named for the objects, plants, or animals they seem to resemble—are believed to help maintain physical well-being and treat disease. A sampling of poses, which should be tried only under trained supervision, appears here.

Increased energy and proper body alignment are the benefits thought to be gained from the dog pose (above), one of the basic standing asanas.

The standing triangle (right) is said to tone the calf, hamstring, and back muscles, and to invigorate the abdominal organs.

The challenging half-bound-lotus forward bend (below) supposedly provides an internal massage to the pelvic region, relieving cramping.

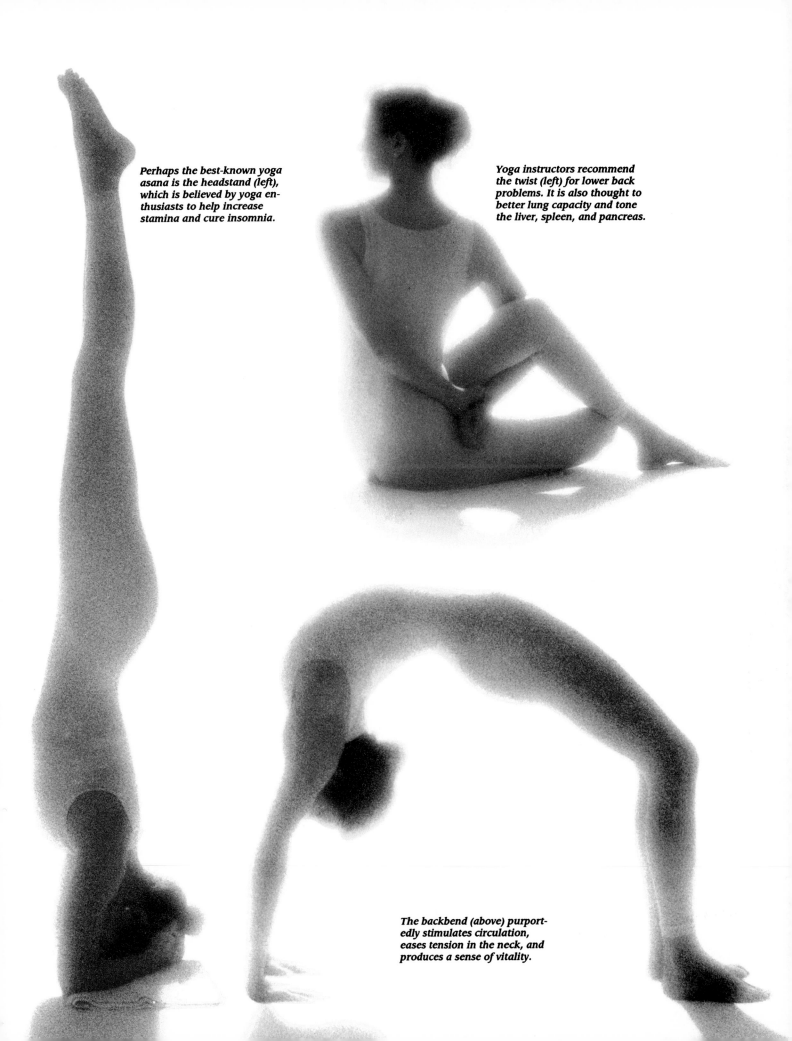

Perhaps the best-known yoga asana is the headstand (left), which is believed by yoga enthusiasts to help increase stamina and cure insomnia.

Yoga instructors recommend the twist (left) for lower back problems. It is also thought to better lung capacity and tone the liver, spleen, and pancreas.

The backbend (above) purportedly stimulates circulation, eases tension in the neck, and produces a sense of vitality.

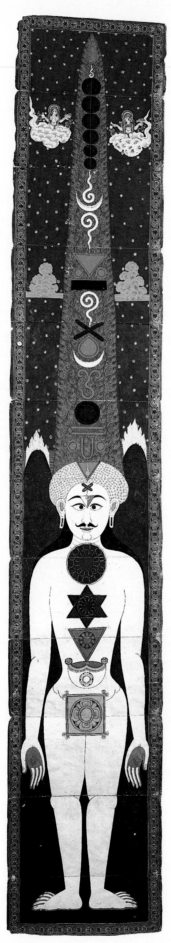

Yoga is mentioned in the Vedas, which it predates, and expounded in some detail in the Upanishads. The specifics of raja-yoga, the philosophical approach dealing most directly with mental and physical health, were collected by the Vedic sage Patanjali in the Yoga Sutras, believed to have been written in the third century BC. Health, however, is not the primary intent of any form of Yoga, whose name literally means "joining." Its ultimate goal is the blissful reuniting of the individual with Brahman—God—the beginning and end of all things, the only true and unchanging reality. Yoga perceives the manifest world as maya—illusion, a deception reflecting humanity's ignorance of its true source, nature, and destiny. Reunion with God ends the illusion and halts the painful round of reincarnations, whose sole purpose is to educate and prepare the soul to return to its true home.

Yoga lays out four main paths to this end: karma-yoga, involving selfless acts; bhakti-yoga, the prayerful worship of God; jnana-yoga, the rigorous exercise of intellect and will; and raja-yoga, which seeks to transform physical energy into spiritual energy through physical and mental discipline. Raja, and a subdivision of it that is called hatha, are probably the Yogic forms best known in the West.

Ayurveda and Yoga, both firmly grounded in India, developed along separate but parallel lines and share certain commonalities. Yogic attitudes toward diet, for instance, echo Ayurvedic tenets. But Yoga, wholly mystical (and sometimes magical) in its orientation, is not a medical system in the same sense as the philosophically based but more pragmatic Ayurveda. Nevertheless, since Yoga considers a sound body an asset on the avenue to spiritual enlightenment, it has, over the centuries, devised its own philosophy of fitness and its own disciplines to help maintain health.

Perhaps the most significant Yogic contribution to oriental healing lore is the idea of prana, a cosmic energy that enters the body with the breath. The concept of prana led to the practice of *pranayama*, breath control, which made its way into Ayurveda.

Prana as a life force is similar to the Chinese idea of qi. And, like qi, prana is thought to flow through an invisible network of tubes, called, in this case, *nadis*. Yoga teaches that the material body is surrounded by a sort of spirit double called the subtle body. Usually, it is said, this entity can be sensed only by the Yoga adept, called a yogi, after long practice, although there are reports of laypeople experiencing it spontaneously. Supposedly, it is this subtle body that contains the nadis. Prana is the vital, animating link between the spiritual self, which survives death and goes on to reincarnation, and the material self, which dies. In a mystical sense, the two bodies are separate. Regarded anatomically, however, they have exact correspondences and operate as one in a living human being. (In China, a similar concept involves the *hun* body, which travels to the next world, and the *po*, which dies. Nevertheless, the energy-bearing meridians run through the actual physical body.)

Like qi, prana is thought to bring health and vitality when it flows freely through the nadis, infusing the body with energy and ridding it of impurities. Prana can also be con-

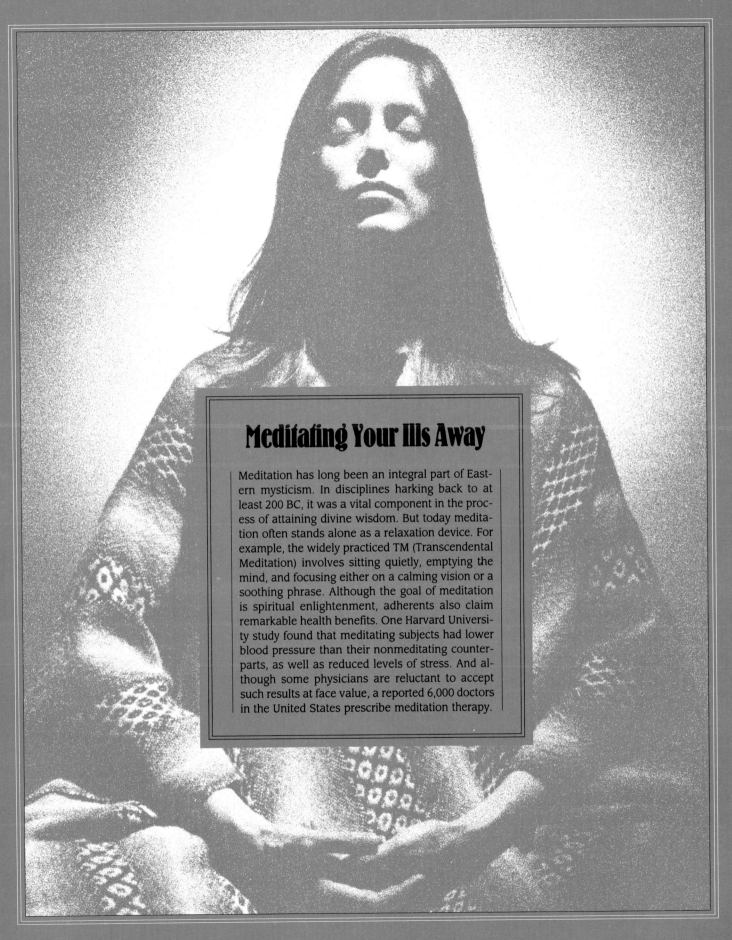

Meditating Your Ills Away

Meditation has long been an integral part of Eastern mysticism. In disciplines harking back to at least 200 BC, it was a vital component in the process of attaining divine wisdom. But today meditation often stands alone as a relaxation device. For example, the widely practiced TM (Transcendental Meditation) involves sitting quietly, emptying the mind, and focusing either on a calming vision or a soothing phrase. Although the goal of meditation is spiritual enlightenment, adherents also claim remarkable health benefits. One Harvard University study found that meditating subjects had lower blood pressure than their nonmeditating counterparts, as well as reduced levels of stress. And although some physicians are reluctant to accept such results at face value, a reported 6,000 doctors in the United States prescribe meditation therapy.

trolled and stored through the breath control of pranayama. The aim of control is to rid the mind of distractions—the mood-induced irregularities in breathing that normally occur throughout the day—and send healing energy to the internal organs. The goal of storing prana is to maximize its benefits as a giver of health and life.

The body's nadis—some 72,000 of them in classical lore—resolve into three main channels, the *pingala, ida,* and *susumna,* which are associated with Ayurveda's three energies, pitta, vata, and kapha. The pingala opens at the right nostril, the ida on the left. The pingala carries the hot sun energy, while the ida carries cool moon energy. These two nadis, representing conflicting forces, spiral downward around the neutral susumna, which runs up the middle of the spine and partakes of both hot and cold. The susumna, the subtle energy conduit that corresponds to the spinal cord in the material body, is the most important of the nadis. Along its length lie six of the seven chakras, or wheels, the vital energy centers of the subtle body. The seventh chakra covers the crown of the head. The chakras, traditionally depicted as lotuses with varying numbers of petals, correspond to certain colors, emotions, organs, nerve plexuses, and ruling deities. From the bottom, the six susumna chakras are located in the rectal area, near the genitals, behind the navel, at the heart, at the throat, and at the point between the eyebrows.

The lowest chakra is said to be the resting place of kundalini, sleeping cosmic energy that is sometimes depicted as a coiled snake. Some yogis aim to awaken the dormant serpent through pranayama, meditation, and other practices. Once roused, the snake begins to climb along the susumna, piercing each chakra in its course. The "kundalini experience," as it is often called by modern practitioners, is said to entail the vitalization of each chakra and its corresponding elements and organs. Energy flows abundantly and disease is banished. More important for Yoga adepts, each piercing brings with it an expanding consciousness. With the penetration of the crown chakra, the thousand-petaled lotus of the abso-lute, the yogi attains samadhi, the superconscious state of bliss in which illusion is banished and time, space, and causation are transcended.

A true master of Yoga or of Ayurveda, or a sincere follower of the Tao, may well spend a lifetime of study in the effort to understand the manifold nuances and complexities of these ancient and multiform disciplines. Whatever their medical worth or verities—and those matters are still in question in the West—they are, after all, the culmination of thousands of years of thought and experience, by turns abstruse, poetic, and brilliant. And in their very depth and richness lies a problem. All provide certain discrete therapies that may benefit patients without requiring them to immerse themselves in a total, underlying system of thought. Acupuncture, for example, may relieve the pain of arthritis—or so its adherents say—regardless of whether the sufferer studies the Tao or believes in yin and yang. Similarly, a person who changes his diet to incorporate more fiber and less fat will probably enjoy improved health, even without reading the Vedas or Upanishads.

Even so, many disciplines of oriental healing were not meant to stand alone. They are threads in an intricate fabric, and each one is best used in the full context of its own tradition. Samplers who pick and choose at the lavish banquet table of mystical Eastern healing may indeed enjoy certain benefits, physical or spiritual. But, say purist and critic alike, they should not assume that they have absorbed the whole feast.

Moreover, in the West, even the most enthusiastic supporters of the Eastern ways do not contend that they should replace Western medicine or supplant the innumerable benefits that it supplies. Rather, they envision the continuing study of the oriental healing traditions and, perhaps, an eventual blending of the best of East and West. "Those who are wise inquire and search together," said China's legendary Yellow Emperor some 5,000 years ago, "while those who are ignorant and stupid inquire and search apart from each other."

Peering into the Body's Secrets

In 1895, Wilhelm Conrad Röntgen discovered a form of radiant energy that enabled him to "see" bones through flesh. When directed at part of a human body, the radiation was absorbed by dense bone tissue but passed through softer substances such as skin and muscle. Thus, when he aimed the rays through his wife's hand at a photographic plate, the German physicist obtained a shadow image of the hand's skeletal structure. Röntgen gave his discovery a name that reflected its unknown nature: the x-ray.

By making reality of what had been a fantastic dream—looking inside the human body without touching knife to flesh—x-rays revolutionized medicine. Doctors the world over eagerly welcomed the new technology, using it to examine bones and diagnose injuries.

Scientists later learned that Röntgen's enigmatic rays were an extremely shortwave form of electromagnetic radiation. This understanding led to refinement of the images. And in the 1970s, the union of computers and radiology spawned a new breed of imaging devices that Röntgen and his contemporaries would have thought as miraculous as his original discovery. Nowadays, such techniques as nuclear

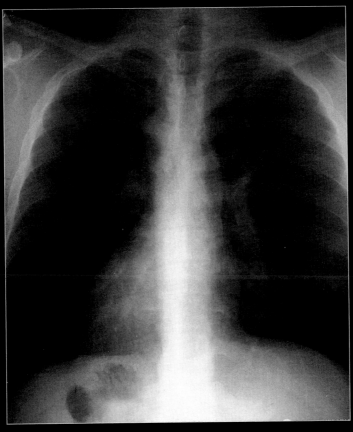

X-ray pictures, such as this one of a healthy man's chest, marked the beginning of conventional medicine's quest for images that open a window into the hidden realms of the body.

magnetic resonance and computerized tomography expose the interior body so detailedly that minute differences in tissue densities are readily visible: An organ can be clearly distinguished from the flesh that surrounds it, and diseased tissue can be distinguished from healthy tissue.

Ironically, the success of scientifically proved techniques has been used as an argument to promote other, highly questionable—some say quackish—diagnostic imaging methods, most notably the ones called radionic and Kirlian photography. Both methods allegedly harness the body's own subtle energies to portray the unseen, instead of relying on an outside force such as radiation. The proponents of radionic photography say it can detect illnesses before physical symptoms ever appear. Endorsers of Kirlian photography count among its advantages the ability to monitor changes in mental as well as physical health.

The medical establishment accepts neither technique; indeed, the distribution of radionic devices for medical purposes has been banned in the United States. Defenders, however, maintain that the methods are efficacious even if not fully understood. They argue, in effect, that since x-rays and computerized image creation do things once thought impossible, their own devices should not be rejected just because scientists say the techniques cannot work.

A closer look at some of the different techniques—orthodox and questionable, approved and unapproved—is presented on the following pages.

Some advocates of Kirlian and radionic photography point to scientifically recognized, advanced medical images as evidence that their own techniques may also someday be accepted by conventional medicine. They argue that their technology may be ahead of its time. It presumes the human body emits a subtle energy field, an assumption mainstream medicine is not ready to adopt. Just so, believers say, traditional doctors a hundred years ago might have been hard put to accept the premises of today's radiology.

Modern imaging devices do create wondrous pictures of the inner body. Nuclear magnetic resonance is often used to view soft tissue, such as the brain. NMR subjects the body to a magnetic field, which is then exposed to a burst of radio waves. That leads to a release of energy signals in a pattern conforming to body tissues.

Computerized tomography is often used to pinpoint tumors. A CAT scanner circles the body with a tightly focused x-ray beam. Then a computer assembles the resulting information to produce a revealing image of a cross-sectional slice.

Thermography uses body temperature to detect malignancies and confirm the presence of pain. When blood flow increases or decreases in part of the body—due to injury, for instance—the temperature of the adjacent skin varies accordingly. Thermographic infrared cameras detect the body's subtle heat emissions and convert them into color-coded images. The body's temperature patterns are usually symmetrical. Asymmetric patches of heat or cold may signal a problem area.

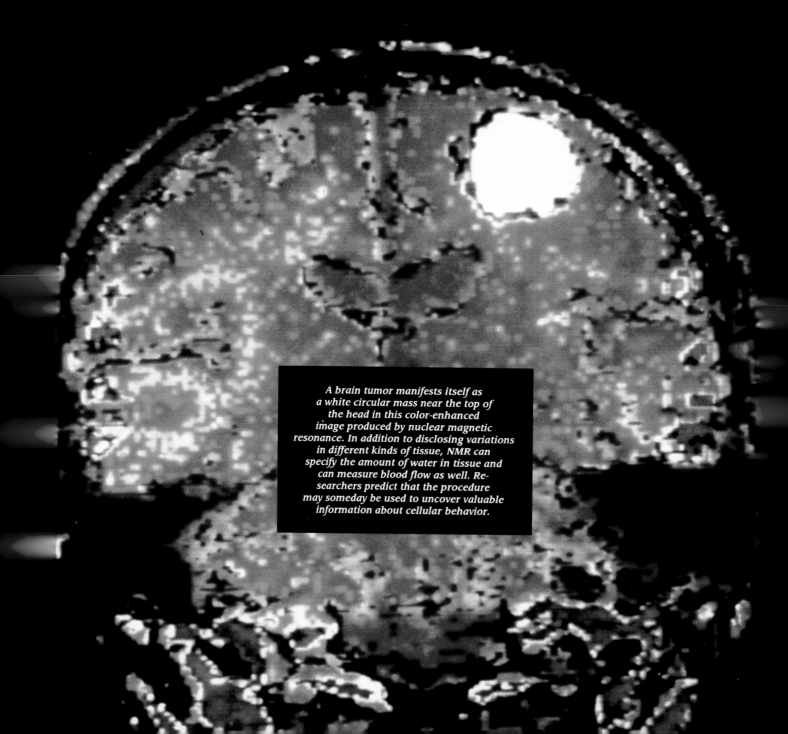

A brain tumor manifests itself as a white circular mass near the top of the head in this color-enhanced image produced by nuclear magnetic resonance. In addition to disclosing variations in different kinds of tissue, NMR can specify the amount of water in tissue and can measure blood flow as well. Researchers predict that the procedure may someday be used to uncover valuable information about cellular behavior.

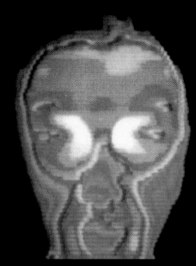

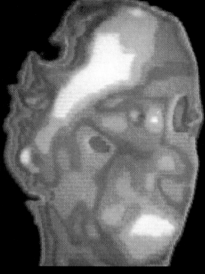

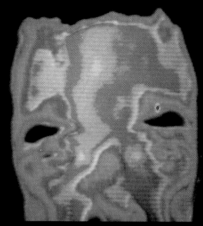

The thermogram above shows the symmetrical temperature patterns that are present in a healthy human head. Colors reflect the subtle heat emissions of the body: White is the hottest, blue is the coolest, and red is intermediate.

The temporal artery, warmer and larger than usual, glows white over the right eye of a migraine sufferer (above). Deviations in temperature pattern, rather than absolute temperature, indicate that there are problem areas in the body.

The asymmetric region of red hues, or relatively cool temperatures, near the left eye signals a trouble spot. Here the telltale aberration is caused by the constricted vessels and reduced blood flow of an extremely painful cluster headache.

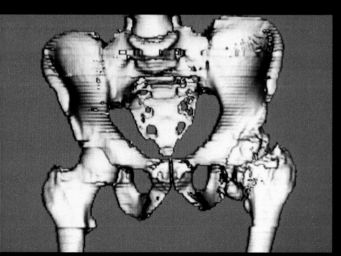

The three-dimensional computerized tomography display above, created from dozens of CAT scans, portrays with great accuracy the affected left hip of a man afflicted with degenerative joint disease. Detailed images such as this one, which can indicate tissue contrast differences as small as a fraction of a percent, have been found to be particularly valuable in the planning of reconstructive surgery.

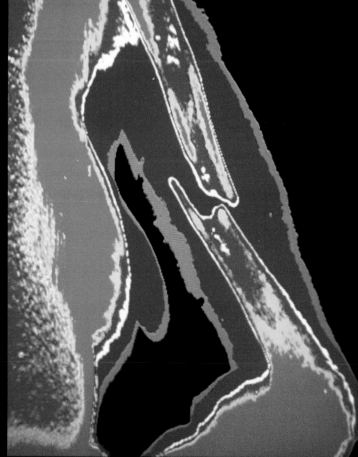

A computerized x-ray (right) vividly exposes the jagged fracture of a young woman's arm bone, which is outlined in white. The color-enhanced image also differentiates tissue densities, permitting a more thorough scrutiny of the injury.

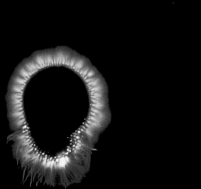
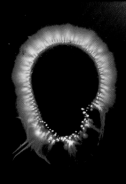

Fiery pink lights illuminate the Kirlian auras of a healer's fingertips at the moment of healing (below). The difference between the healing auras and the more subdued coronas of rest (above) supposedly reflects the energy being emitted.

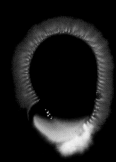
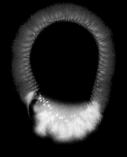

In the late 1950s, the Soviet husband-and-wife team of Semyon and Valentina Kirlian published their research on a fascinating method of imaging: a photographic process capturing a normally invisible energy field, or bioenergy, that they said radiates from every living organism. The technique involved placing an object or part of the body directly on film laid atop a metal plate, which was then subjected to a high-voltage current. A distinct pattern showed around the object in the developed picture. This was assumed to be the bioenergy, or aura. The Kirlians said an individual's biological state, including disease, could be judged by studying auras.

Kirlian photography supposedly discloses emotional information as well: The auras of a healthy, calm person appear to differ from those of an anxious, tense subject. Moreover, some researchers believe that Kirlian photographs can show psychic interaction, especially between individuals with reputed healing powers and their patients.

Scientists say physiological variations at the surface of the skin—such as moisture, temperature, and pressure—produce the differences in the "auras." They further explain that the image on film is actually that of a corona discharge in a gas, a natural electrical phenomenon.

Thelma Moss of UCLA, a leading pioneer of American research into Kirlian photography, has countered by arguing that even if the phenomenon is a corona discharge, the changes that occur in it under varying conditions make it worthy of study. In a 1978 report, Rumanian researchers asserted that cancer tumors photograph differently than normal tissue. They purportedly detected breast cancer with 100 percent accuracy through Kirlian methods. Alfred Benjamin in Los Angeles reported that his research indicated that blood from cancer victims displayed a Kirlian aura different from that produced by blood from people who did not have cancer. One medical research team in the early 1980s found the technique promising in the possible diagnosis of asthma. The hand coronas, or auras, of people with the condition tended to display a distinctive wispy pattern. Such results have encouraged continued investigation into Kirlian photography.

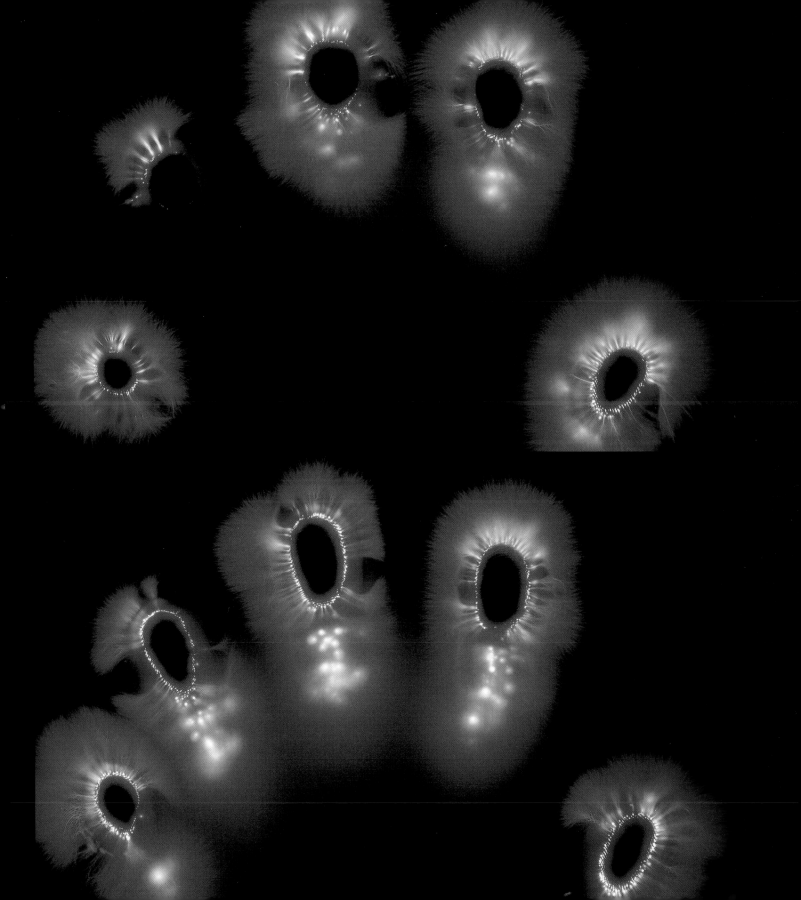

Radionic Pictures of "Vibrational Energies"

Proponents of radionics hail it as a holistic approach to healing. Detractors label it, at best, an offbeat system that depends on the unreliable placebo effect. At worst, it is condemned as potentially dangerous quackery that may delay people from seeking necessary medical care.

Like Kirlian photography, radionics presumes all individuals radiate an invisible energy field. But radionic practitioners stray much further from scientific truths. They claim that a mere blood spot or lock of hair—the "witness"—can transmit a person's "vibrational energies." By placing the witness in a special black box and then stroking a pad connected to the box, the operator supposedly senses the emanations from the substance. He tunes dials on the box and makes a diagnosis from the rates of emanations; then his psychic consciousness sends healing vibrations to the patient. Thus an ailment that may not yet have manifested physical symptoms is cured through radionics.

Dr. Albert Abrams of California invented the first radionic instrument in the early 1900s. In the 1930s, Hollywood chiropractor Ruth Drown declared it possible to treat patients from a distance using the radionic witness. She also developed radionic photography, which purportedly produces images of problem areas in the body via the energy of the witness streaming across film. Drown's work proved controversial: In 1951, she was convicted of medical fraud, and the distribution of her radionic devices was banned by the Food and Drug Administration.

Still, radionics retains its followers, some no doubt charlatans, but others sincere believers who hope the practice may someday transform orthodox medicine.

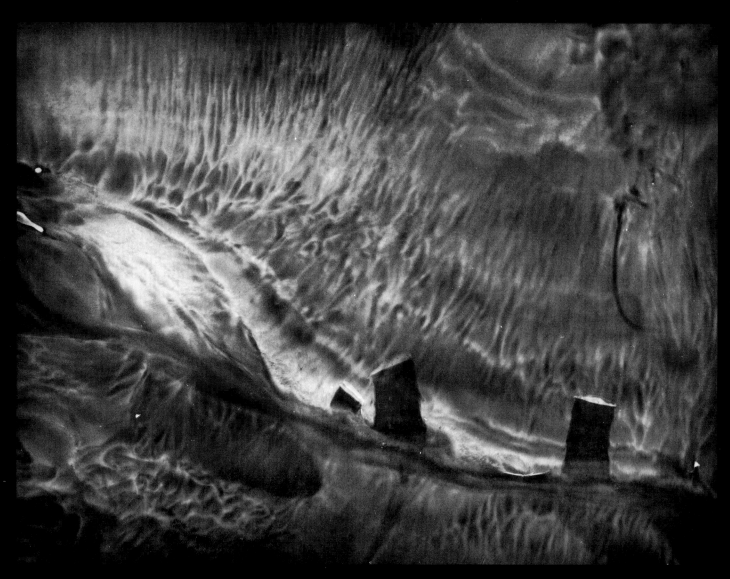

This radionic photograph, obtained at Ruth Drown's laboratory in the 1930s from a blood spot placed in her Radio-Vision camera, supposedly shows an inside view of an abdominal surgery scar. The patient was allegedly a block away when the picture was created.

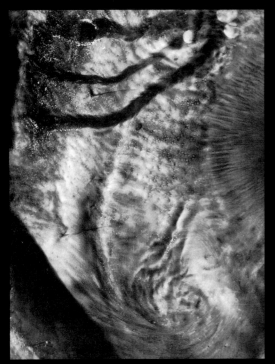 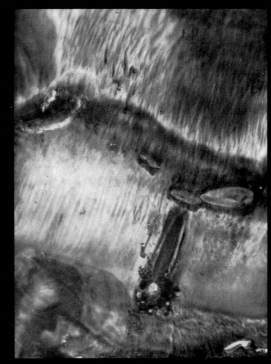

Made in Drown's Hollywood laboratory from the blood spot of a patient residing in Indiana, this radionic photograph ostensibly shows a cancerous section of the liver. The quality of radionic images apparently depends on the psychic skills of the camera operator. The very presence of a skeptic is enough to prevent an image from being obtained, say practitioners.

The tiny white dots in the picture above, taken in Drown's laboratory, purportedly indicate an infection of the lower spine. The problem was detected through radionic methods. Then the camera's dials were tuned in to the emanation rate to produce the picture of the diseased area. Practitioners say training is necessary to interpret most radionic images.

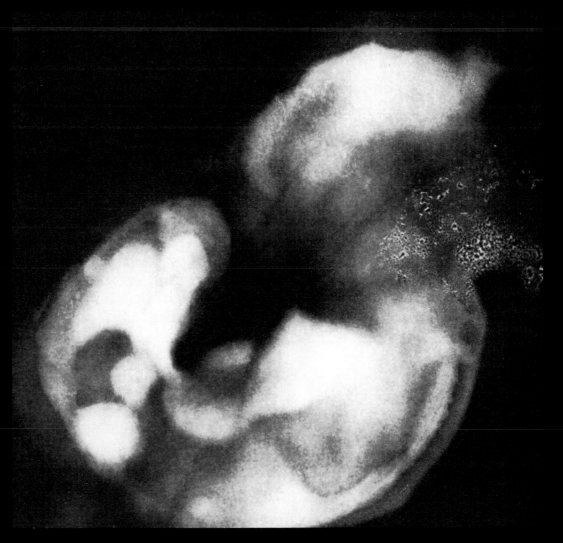

Around 1950, the Delawarr Laboratories located in Oxford, England, produced this radionic photograph, considered to be the image of a three-month-old fetus, from the blood spot of a pregnant woman said to have been fifty-four miles away. Skeptics note that while the image may resemble a fetus, no evidence proves its authenticity. They contend that the power of suggestion leads people to believe that radionic images represent particular conditions.

CHAPTER 3

Faith and the Human Touch

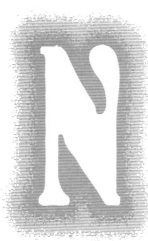

ot long ago in the United States, a baby known only as Benjamin was born virtually without a brain; he had no more than a brainstem, the area at the brain's base that controls the functions of the heart, lungs, and muscles and that normally connects the spinal cord to the higher brain centers. For the brief period that he lived, Benjamin existed in a near vacuum of the senses: He could not see, hear, smell, taste, or think. But when he was picked up and held, he seemed, on some rudimentary level, to sense the holder's touch. Baby Benjamin was deprived of a brain, but he had his skin, and the skin has nerve cells that are connected directly to the spinal cord. Benjamin's sense of touch rescued him from total isolation, from being completely alone in the universe. He could at least feel the arms that held him and the hands that caressed him.

Of all the organs in the human body, the skin is by far the largest and undoubtedly one of the most important. An average adult is clothed in about eighteen square feet of skin, weighing some eight pounds. Spread over this expanse are no fewer than five million tiny, exquisitely sensitive nerve endings, or touch receptors. They reach out to every millimeter of the human envelope, to the delicately translucent eyelids and the tough soles of the feet, to the flavor-exploring tongue, to the nose, the ears, the scalp, and the erogenous zones that stimulate reproduction and thus are crucial to the species' survival. A single fingertip might have 1,000 finely tuned sensors, a hand more than 10,000. In one way or another, the skin's receptors are involved with all of life's touch and taste sensations: soft, hard, sweet, sour, rough, smooth, light, heavy, cold, warm, arousing. They also register the emotional content of touch: the brief, cool brush of disapproval; the hard, hurtful impact of anger; the tentative clutch of anxiety and fear; and the gentle stroke of love or sympathy.

But some people think that the skin's sensors have qualities even more extraordinary than these. It is believed that the receptors transmit real therapeutic power from outside the body to help mend ailments inside. This power is provided by another person: The healing touch is more than just a pleasant turn of phrase.

Hands reaching out to counteract pain with touch is a universal human act, of course. A mother's soothing palm and comforting kiss can do wonders for a child's fevered brow or bruise. A friendly arm around a harried colleague's shoulder may ease a splitting headache. But the therapeutic effect of touch goes far beyond such comforting gestures.

The laying on of hands to effect cures has been accepted by many as a bona fide instrument of healing from the earliest days of humankind. Legend and history and today's news abound with accounts of healers who seem to possess supernormal powers of touch, whose hands can alleviate severe symptoms and complex medical conditions. Healers' hands have been said to drive off disease, to rejuvenate old and crippled bodies, and to restore the ailing to lives of health and happiness. The list of maladies that have been or can be cured by one healing touch or another is nothing short of astonishing, if credited as true—everything from arthritis and asthma to bursitis, cancer, cataracts, cerebral palsy, epilepsy, gallstones, heart disease, paralysis, tuberculosis, vertigo, and tooth decay. Sometimes physical contact is apparently not necessary; many healers, finding that a patient's belief in their power seems of itself to be enough to banish illness, practice at a distance, dispensing with touch entirely.

Down through the ages, different cultures have known those who exercise this seemingly miraculous touch by a variety of names: shamans, witch doctors, strokers, mesmerists, faith healers, magnetic healers, spirit healers, and psychic healers. Many such practitioners have had strong ties to religion. In the West today, quite a few healers—but by no means all—are Christian evangelists. Nowadays, as in the past, healers have difficulty successfully explaining their powers to the world at large. They may speak in terms of God, universal life forces, High Sense Perception, magnetic balance, auras, and energy fields. But exactly how it all works, if it does, remains a general mystery.

Many people contend that such healing does not work at all. And there can be no doubt that out-and-out charlatans as well as honest but ineffective would-be wonderworkers abound among those proclaiming themselves healers. But the practice goes back so far, the reported successes are so widespread and often well-documented, and so many modern-day healers demonstrate a willingness to submit their abilities to the scrutiny of orthodox science and medicine that their sincerity is recognized and their alleged powers are being carefully examined.

The laying on of hands as a form of medicine dates back at least 15,000 years, to the period when Stone Age artists carved into the walls of Pyrenean caves pictographs of

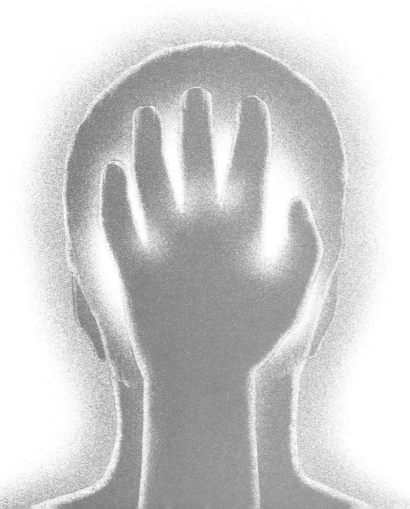

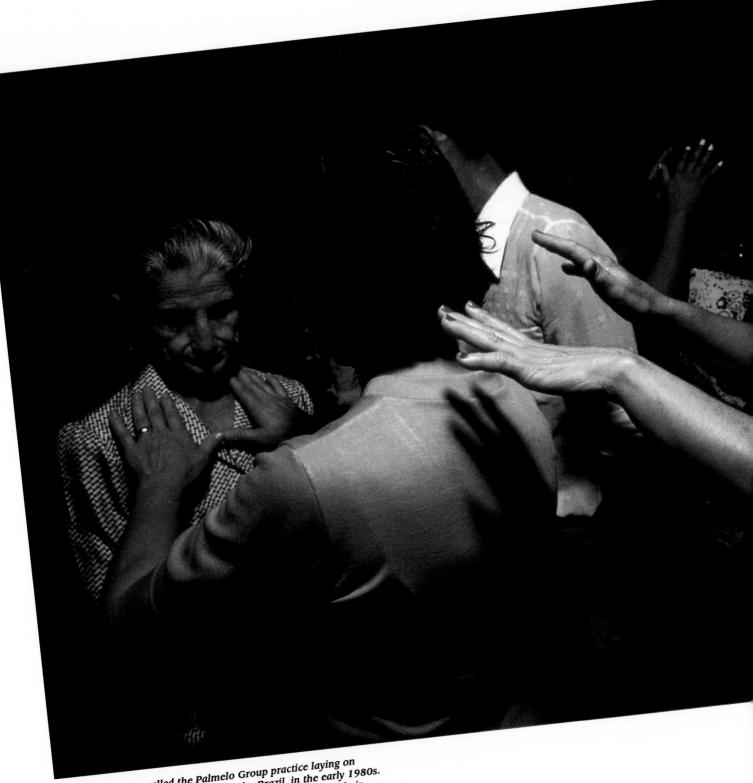

Members of a sect called the Palmelo Group practice laying on
of hands at a healing session in Palmelo, Brazil, in the early 1980s.
Followers believe that divine healing energy flows through their
hands, enabling them not only to effect miraculous cures in those
individuals that they touch, but to exorcise evil spirits as well.

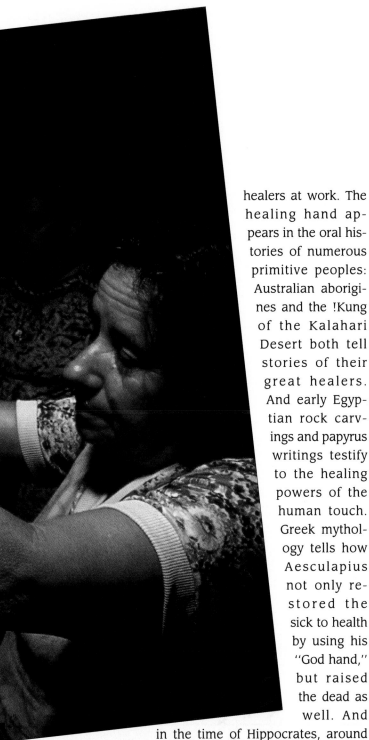

healers at work. The healing hand appears in the oral histories of numerous primitive peoples: Australian aborigines and the !Kung of the Kalahari Desert both tell stories of their great healers. And early Egyptian rock carvings and papyrus writings testify to the healing powers of the human touch. Greek mythology tells how Aesculapius not only restored the sick to health by using his "God hand," but raised the dead as well. And in the time of Hippocrates, around 400 BC, Greek *cheirourgos* (whence the term *surgeon*) ministered not primarily with scalpels, but with healing palms and fingers. One member of the Hippocratic school in Cos wrote that he often was able to alleviate his patients' symptoms "by laying my hands on, or moving them over, the area concerned, as if my hands possessed some strange healing power."

Among the Romans, the renowned Galen, physician to the emperor Marcus Aurelius in the second century AD, fol-lowed Hippocrates' example by employing gentle massage as a healing method. Nor were physicians the only healers. Various Roman emperors were said to have a strong healing touch. Hadrian was reputedly able to relieve dropsy by a laying on of royal hands, while Vespasian was noted for his cures of neurological disorders, as well as lameness and blindness. They were no match, however, for an earlier pagan monarch, King Pyrrhus of Epirus, who in the third century BC was famed for curing colic by the laying on not of hands, but of toes. Hands, toes, or whatever, the royal healing touch was an apparently divine gift that would continue through the ages until well into the eighteenth century.

The New Testament describes how Jesus touched blind eyes (or treated them with his spittle) and restored sight, touched crippled legs and made them strong again, touched ruined heads and brought them back to sanity. The unfortunate came daily and in multitudes, as Luke attested: "Now when the sun was setting, all they that had any sick with divers diseases brought them unto him; and he laid his hands on every one of them and healed them."

Matthew quotes Jesus specifically instructing the apostles to carry on after him: "Heal the sick, raise the dead, cleanse the lepers, cast out devils." Following Christ's command, the disciples regarded their duty to heal to be as important as preaching. One day when a lame beggar accosted Peter and John, Peter answered the piteous pleas for alms with the words: "Silver and Gold I have none, but in the name of Jesus Christ of Nazareth stand up and walk." Whereupon Peter lifted the beggar to his feet "and immediately his feet and ankle bones received strength. And he leaping up, stood, and walked, and entered with them into the Temple, walking and leaping and praising God."

Later Christians—among them Saints Francis, Augustine, Ambrose, Martin, Catherine, Patrick, and Bernard—all were renowned for their healing touch. And like Jesus, the Christian saints attended to illnesses of the mind as well as the body. The story is told of a day in the fourth century when a distraught father brought his son to the saintly hermit Macarius, living in the Egyptian desert. The boy was

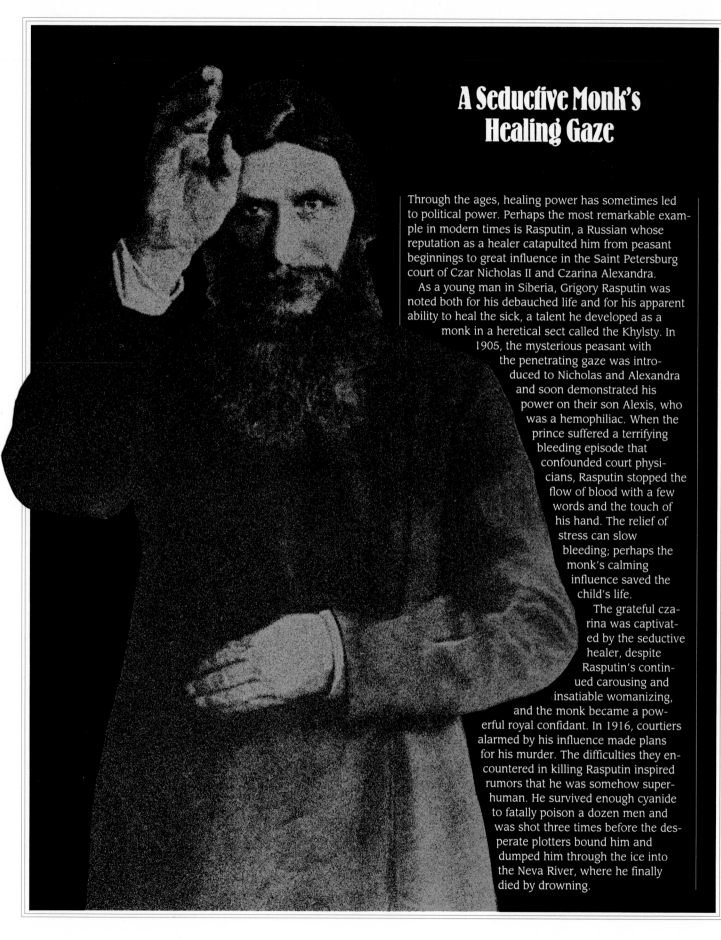

A Seductive Monk's Healing Gaze

Through the ages, healing power has sometimes led to political power. Perhaps the most remarkable example in modern times is Rasputin, a Russian whose reputation as a healer catapulted him from peasant beginnings to great influence in the Saint Petersburg court of Czar Nicholas II and Czarina Alexandra.

As a young man in Siberia, Grigory Rasputin was noted both for his debauched life and for his apparent ability to heal the sick, a talent he developed as a monk in a heretical sect called the Khylsty. In 1905, the mysterious peasant with the penetrating gaze was introduced to Nicholas and Alexandra and soon demonstrated his power on their son Alexis, who was a hemophiliac. When the prince suffered a terrifying bleeding episode that confounded court physicians, Rasputin stopped the flow of blood with a few words and the touch of his hand. The relief of stress can slow bleeding; perhaps the monk's calming influence saved the child's life.

The grateful czarina was captivated by the seductive healer, despite Rasputin's continued carousing and insatiable womanizing, and the monk became a powerful royal confidant. In 1916, courtiers alarmed by his influence made plans for his murder. The difficulties they encountered in killing Rasputin inspired rumors that he was somehow superhuman. He survived enough cyanide to fatally poison a dozen men and was shot three times before the desperate plotters bound him and dumped him through the ice into the Neva River, where he finally died by drowning.

thought to be possessed by evil spirits. Macarius placed his hands upon the boy, one hand on his head and the other on his heart, and commenced to pray. The youth's body gradually became more and more swollen. At last, he gave a cry, and an immense amount of water poured from him, after which his body returned to normal. He was cured.

The Christian tradition of miraculous cures continued throughout the Middle Ages and into the Renaissance. Along with human touch, all manner of sanctified objects—relics that were touched by or were the remains of the holy—were seen to have an effect: bits of the True Cross, scraps of bread from the Last Supper, the shrouds, skulls, bones, and hair reputedly belonging to saints. One sixteenth-century German collector claimed to have amassed 17,000 holy relics—which inspired Pope Leo X to calculate that such piety had saved the man exactly 694,779,550½ days in purgatory.

As in earlier times, those who claimed a divine right to rule were also credited with a divine power to heal. Goiter and scrofula, a tubercular inflammation of the lymph nodes, were common ailments of the day, and the royal touch seemed particularly effective against them. Robert the Pious of France and Edward the Confessor of England reportedly cured such afflictions by placing their hands on the necks of the sick and making the sign of the cross. Such were the royal powers that a king could merely touch an object to impart healing. Henry VIII would touch rings and give them to epileptics, while Charles II is reputed to have passed out 90,798 gold coins to the sick. There is some question as to whether Charles gave the coins or whether he sold them to his patients.

There were touch healers among the commonfolk as well. Known as *chiothetists,* they were much respected in the countryside until 1423 when the English Guild of Physicians denounced them as "quacks and empirics and knavish men and women," after which they fell into decline. Yet in later years there was a commoner, albeit a wealthy one, whose healing abilities rivaled in fame those of the royals. He was Valentine Greatrakes, a seventeenth-century Irish landowner and magistrate, who practiced a technique known as stroking. Greatrakes began by placing his hands on the ill person's head, sometimes gently rubbing it. Then he would stroke the ailment downward three times "until the pain," as he put it, "were driven out the toes' ends." Describing the effect on a crippled seaman, Greatrakes boasted that the man "walked lustily to and fro in the garden, professing his willingness to do so for ten miles, and carrying the crutches—sometimes in his hand, sometimes triumphantly on his shoulders—which had previously supported him."

No less a personage than Robert Boyle, the founder of modern chemistry, testified to Greatrakes's success. And in 1666, the healer embarked on a highly successful tour of London, taking on cases of paralysis, deafness, headache, and arthritis, for which he would accept no payment. But the medical establishment paid him no heed, and skeptics argued that it was mainly a matter of illusion. As one contemporary account put it: "So great was the confidence in him, that the blind fancied they saw the light which they could not see, the deaf imagined that they heard, the lame that they walked straight and the paralytic that they had recovered the use of their limbs." Eventually, the skeptics won out. Greatrakes quietly returned to his estate in Ireland and gave up the practice of healing.

Even at the pinnacle of his popularity, Valentine Greatrakes could not match an eighteenth-century Parisian by the name of Franz Anton Mesmer. Born in Austria in 1734, Mesmer had studied both philosophy and law before entering the University of Vienna for a doctorate in medicine. Energetic and charming, he had attracted a wealthy wife and the friendship of such notables as Mozart even before receiving his degree, and once in practice, he quickly became known in his own right.

Formulating fresh theories about health and illness, Mesmer argued that there was a universal fluid, a sort of life force, that permeated the cosmos and everything in it. Human illness was the result of an imbalance or blockage of

Electrifying Aids to Health

In the middle of the eighteenth century, the blossoming study of electricity gripped the public imagination of the Western world as no science had before. The enigmatic energy proved as entertaining as it was intriguing; newly invented static electricity generators soon found their way into parlor games, where guests' hair was made to stand literally on end. From such amusements, as well as from more sober investigation, grew early attempts to use electricity in the medical treatment of paralysis, hysteria, and exhaustion.

By the end of the century, however, the mysterious powers of electricity were being turned to what some considered darker purposes. A British surgeon, Charles Kite, invented a primitive cardiac defibrillator, which could restart a recently stilled heart with a jolt of electricity. This and other electrical devices employed in attempts to revive the dead were perceived by many as the devil's work. Tainted thus with the occult, as well as by an alleged association with mesmerism, the once-promising phenomenon lost credibility with most doctors.

In a photograph from the early 1860s, Guillaume Duchenne touches an electrode to a patient who has no feeling in his face—just one of the French physician's pioneering experiments exploring the effects of electrical stimulation on diseased nerves and muscles.

In 1858, a Philadelphia dentist named Jerome Francis patented a method of "painless tooth extraction by electromagnetism," using a generator like the one above. One wire led to a metal handle held by the patient. The other was attached to the dental forceps and delivered a current that temporarily deadened feeling around the tooth.

A drawing of a man trussed by a Pulvermacher Electric Belt (right) illustrates how the popular nineteenth-century device was to be worn. Falsely touted as a cure-all, the belt was a string of very small batteries that generated a weak electrical current after being soaked in vinegar.

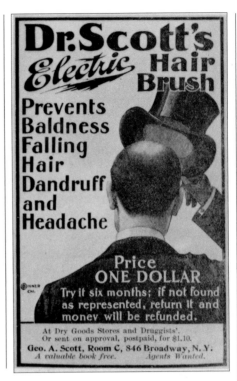

The study of electrical science nonetheless continued to advance. More sophisticated generating devices were invented. And by the mid-1800s, the work of European physiologists such as Guillaume Duchenne—who studied the effect of electrical stimulation on nerves and muscles—revived medical interest in electricity by elucidating the function it performed in the body.

Public attention soon followed suit, with Americans in particular looking to electrotherapy as a means of easing human suffering. Numerous electrical devices for curing various aches and ailments appeared on the market and were eagerly bought by the hopeful—and the curious. Some of the products did have therapeutic potential. Others, such as "electric" liniments, rings, and brushes were electric in name only and obviously the work of charlatans. Early in the twentieth century, this element of quackery again caused physicians to abandon their interest in electrotherapy.

In recent years, however, electricity has regained its reputation as a valuable medical tool. Indeed, some modern devices, such as electrical nerve stimulators to relieve pain and cardiac pacemakers, hark back to eighteenth- and nineteenth-century predecessors. And as for the once-ominous practice of reviving the dead—electrical resuscitation devices are now standard equipment in emergency rooms.

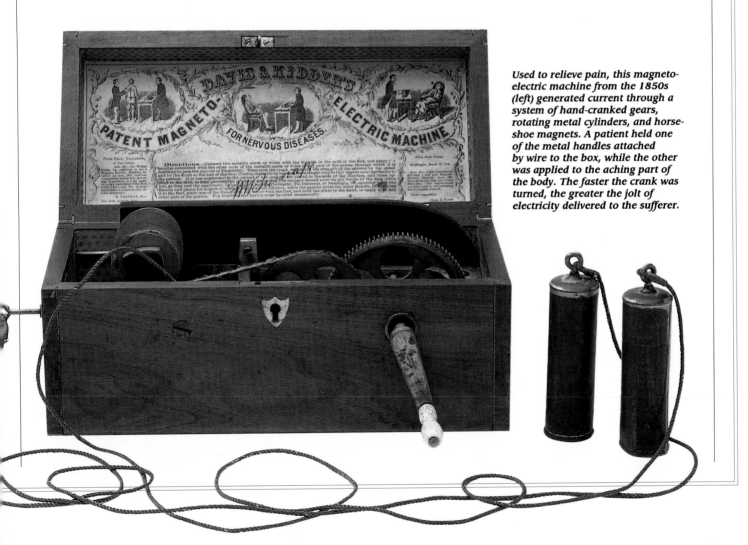

Used to relieve pain, this magneto-electric machine from the 1850s (left) generated current through a system of hand-cranked gears, rotating metal cylinders, and horseshoe magnets. A patient held one of the metal handles attached by wire to the box, while the other was applied to the aching part of the body. The faster the crank was turned, the greater the jolt of electricity delivered to the sufferer.

fluid in the body. In this, Mesmer may have been borrowing from the ancient traditions of prana in India and qi in China, which postulated a universal energy in control of all life: When the energy was balanced and flowing unhindered, good health resulted; an impeded energy flow meant sickness and disease.

Mesmer believed his universal fluid to be magnetic in nature and termed it animal magnetism. He theorized that polarized magnetic forces kept the fluid in balance and coursing through healthy bodies and that magnetic forces could reestablish balance and flow in unhealthy ones.

In Vienna and later in Paris, the doctor claimed to restore his patients' essential polarity by touching them with a slender iron wand about ten inches in length; some individuals he touched with his hands or simply fixed with a penetrating gaze, the look of which was enough to establish a rapport, as he called it. His manipulations of animal magnetism over the patient's body brought on crises, as he termed them, that were a vital part of the healing process. These muscle spasms and seizures, frequently accompanied by wild singing, screaming, and raving, eventually waned, and the patient regained a normal equilibrium. Mesmer regarded his patients as cured when his ministrations no longer brought on crises.

Mesmer's patients, who included some of the richest and most prominent figures in Paris, were afflicted with ailments ranging from asthma to blindness, deafness, migraine headaches, and paralysis, along with a wide variety of internal disorders. One who wrote specifically of his cure was an army major, the chevalier de Haussay, who had endured years of ill health stemming from frostbite suffered on campaign in Hanover and malignant fever contracted in Martinique. When he went to see Mesmer, he staggered, stuttered (when he could speak at all), and trembled uncontrollably; his eyes bulged unnaturally from their sockets, and he lapsed into fits of hysterical laughter. Mesmer's treatments produced a series of shuddering convulsions, reported de Haussay, "ice coming from my limbs, followed by great heat and foetid perspiration. Now, after four months, I am completely cured."

The healer's wealthiest disciples paid to learn the Austrian's secrets. So great was his following that in 1784, Louis XVI set up a royal commission to investigate Mesmer's methods and results. Among its distinguished members were Benjamin Franklin, the American ambassador, and a certain Dr. Joseph-Ignace Guillotin, who won lasting fame by inventing a "painless beheading machine" just in time for the French Revolution. The commission spent six months looking into mesmerism before reaching their verdict: "The magnetic field could not be perceived by any of the senses, and its existence could not be inferred from any effects observed either in themselves or in any of the patients examined." The commission concluded that Mesmer's apparent cures were due to the patients' susceptible imaginations and not to any so-called animal magnetism.

There it all rested for many years. Mesmer faded from the scene, but his healing ideas continued to evolve in the work of others. Among his most ardent disciples were two aristocrats, the marquis de Puységur and his brother, Count Maxime. They were the first to examine the effects of mesmerism on the mind and to observe that a mesmerized patient would obey the instructions of the mesmerist. Their efforts, in effect, identified what would later be termed the subconscious mind and the process known as hypnosis.

Nineteenth-century American society was in turbulent flux. The frontiers of science, industry, and popular culture were wide open to new ideas. While intellectuals experimented with Utopian communities, the growing middle class tried out fresh philosophies at meetings in lecture halls, opera houses, and Chautauqua tents. Traditional churches were hard-pressed to reconcile the new notions with fundamental Biblical precepts, and bewildered congregations sought a spiritual understanding of where they belonged in this era of upheaval and change.

Interest in Spiritualism and the occult was rampant, and charismatic faith healers such as Andrew Jackson Davis

Europe's Healer of Thousands

Serge Léon Alalouf professed to cure only those who truly believed in his power of touch. If so, then the faithful numbered at least 276,000, for that many testimonial letters arrived at a Paris courthouse in 1957, when Alalouf was accused—and acquitted—of unlawfully practicing medicine.

Alalouf, born in 1905, claimed he first recognized his healing gift when, as a young man in Toulouse, he touched a man's badly wounded head and within days the injury disappeared. In over fifty years of practice, the darkly handsome healer counted among his clientele King Alfonso XIII of Spain and French playwright Jean Anouilh. Alalouf also may have been clairvoyant: After predicting a violent end for himself, the healer was killed by an automobile in 1982.

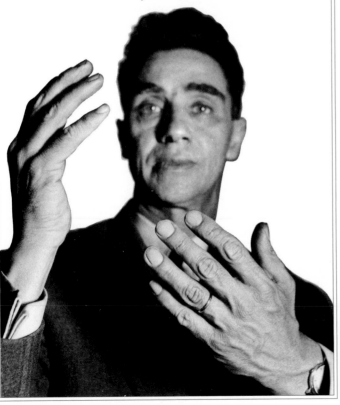

in New York and J. R. Newton in Rhode Island held mass meetings to demonstrate their skills. Crowds came as much for entertainment as for therapy. Davis, a cobbler from Poughkeepsie, drew from Mesmer's ideas for what he called his harmonial philosophy and recorded his successful work in thirty books. Newton, in the name of Christian love, employed a variety of techniques. He poured hot water over the heads of patients with nervous disorders but opted for a simple laying on of hands to treat tumors or swellings.

Another New England healer, Phineas Parkhurst Quimby of Portland, Maine, started out using mesmerism and magnetic sweeps of the body in treating his patients. But as his practice grew, he began to suspect that what really cured people was neither divine intervention nor the way he manipulated their animal magnetism, but how he changed their mental attitudes toward their ailments.

Quimby believed that the faith his patients had in his ability to help them was as important as any other factor. He came to see the mind as the key agent of healing, and he thought that if he could convince a patient that a disease was actually caused by mental attitude, the explanation would effect a cure; the patient's understanding would draw the body's energy fluids into healthy balance.

In 1862, Quimby agreed to see a Massachusetts woman who had written to him about her spinal problems. By the time she arrived at his office in Portland, she was so crippled that she had to be carried into his waiting room. She was forty-one years old and had already appealed unsuccessfully to physicians and homeopaths. Nevertheless, with mesmerism, gentle massage, and a great deal of calming talk, Quimby relieved her condition—and won a devoted follower. That patient would eventually become famous as Mary Baker Eddy, the founder of the Christian Science faith, whose tenets owe much to her close study of Quimby's work *(pages 124-125)*.

The Church of Christ, Scientist, is by no means the only vehicle by which faith and religion have come to play a strong role in twentieth-century healing. A multitude of modern-day healers from many different sects regard them-

Hypnosis: The Drugless Anesthetic

Working within the intangible realms of the unconscious mind, hypnosis relieves many people of very real bodily pain. After hypnotic induction, for instance, some patients face the dentist's drill armed with only the suggestion of numbness. Women in childbirth forgo drugs and rely instead on hypnotic techniques to cope. And cancer patients often require less pain medication after hypnosis—in the bargain gaining a therapeutic sense of control over the ravaging disease.

Such victories over pain are possible because hypnosis alters the way a person actually feels physical stimuli: Suggestions made to the unconscious mind of an individual in a hypnotic trance apparently distort the perceptions of the conscious mind. For instance, in one study a hypnotized man was told that he would be touched with a cold wire. When instead a hot wire was put to his skin, he reportedly experienced no pain.

Responsiveness to hypnotic suggestion varies from one person to another. Trust in the hypnotist also influences the depth of a trance—and thus the degree of pain relief. Motivation has been found to affect susceptibility to hypnosis as well: An unusually high proportion of burn victims achieve substantial control over their suffering through hypnosis, perhaps because they are desperate for respite from excruciating pain.

Any number of techniques can be used to bring pain under control. After inducing hypnosis, the therapist may suggest that part of the body will become so numb that no pain can be felt in it. Or a patient might be asked to imagine that a sore arm, for instance, no longer belongs to him.

In another method, a patient is told to make a fist, to imagine capturing all the pain in it, and then to throw that pain away. Still another technique invokes a patient's memory, suggesting that he or she relive an earlier, pain-free experience to block out current suffering.

Some dentists, in particular, have found hypnosis useful. "With the mind at rest, and total muscular relaxation, everything goes more smoothly," says English dentist Ian Wilkie. He claims that through hypnotism he can drill and fill the teeth of most children and some adults without anesthetic—and without pain. When a procedure does require a painkiller, he says, a smaller-than-usual dose does the job.

Although hypnosis is rarely used as the sole anesthetic during surgery— few people can suppress pain entirely—it has proved valuable in relaxing a patient before a procedure and in reducing postoperative pain. Additionally, the reassurance hypnosis imparts may speed healing: Confident patients tend to recover sooner than anxious ones.

Some studies have shown that hypnosis enables the mind to help heal the body in more direct ways. For instance, a hypnotized patient can reportedly reduce bleeding from a tooth extraction by imagining the blood flow is turned off like water from a faucet. And some skin diseases and allergic conditions, such as hay fever, improve in response to hypnosis. Since such ailments are often linked to anxiety, the relaxation element of hypnosis probably accounts for the cure.

Some attribute the pain-controlling abilities of hypnosis mainly to relaxation—mixed, perhaps, with some stoicism and even a little fakery by the patient. Most researchers, however, believe hypnotic suggestion truly alters pain perception at the higher levels of the nervous system. And although the physiology of the sleeplike condition remains a mystery, the pain relief it grants many is clear; indeed, the American Medical Association endorsed hypnosis as a means of controlling pain as far back as 1958.

Dentist Ian Wilkie, who employs chemical painkillers only as a supplement to hypnotic suggestion, prepares to treat a patient.

selves as instruments of God, chosen to transmit divine power by means of touch or the laying on of hands, and through prayer, songs, meditation, and visualization.

Healers can be found in virtually every Christian denomination in America. One well-known twentieth-century healer was Olga Worrall, a member of the Methodist laity, who with her husband, Ambrose, began practicing in 1950 at Baltimore's Mt. Washington United Methodist Church. The Worralls believed that their power was a direct gift from God. Mrs. Worrall first suspected that she was specially chosen when she was only three years old, when one day her mother complained of a headache. The little girl touched the woman's forehead, and according to the story, the headache instantly disappeared. Olga said her parents acknowledged her gift but played it down because they did not want her regarded as a freak.

She met her husband at a college dance and in time realized that he was gifted as well. Yet it was not until they were in their forties that they gave serious attention to healing through their church. The Thursday morning sessions at the Mt. Washington church were simple ceremonies. There were pews for only about 300 people, and they were usually full. The church's minister was always in attendance. Mrs. Worrall would address the assembly first, explaining that there was no guarantee that anyone would be healed. "We have had cases that are like miracles. We've had others that have been greatly helped. And we've had others that were untouched," she said at one service. "Why? I don't know—and that's mostly because it is not I who heals, but the spiritual power that comes from God. I put my hands on you and pray, but it is God who does the work."

She went on to explain that there would be no charge for their help and that—she stressed this point—she and her husband fully endorsed orthodox medicine. They would treat only people who already were under a physician's care. Next came an interlude of organ music, the minister's brief sermon, and some hymn singing. Then all those who wished help would be invited to come forward and kneel for a laying on of hands. Olga or Ambrose Worrall would greet a supplicant and inquire about the problem, then lay on hands if that seemed appropriate, pray for two or three minutes, and finally murmur "God bless you" before turning to the next person. When everyone had been ministered to, all who wanted to linger shared lunch in the parish hall.

Those who had been touched, particularly those who had felt Olga Worrall's hands, described a powerful sensation of heat infusing their bodies. Mrs. Worrall herself characterized her hands during healing as feeling warm, as though they were heating pads; she often experienced an electric tingling as well.

Whatever the physical sensations, the Worralls were credited with some amazing results. In their 1965 book *The Gift of Healing*, there appeared a number of testimonials to the couple's healing powers. One letter written by a surgeon involved a woman with a cancerous tumor in her abdomen. According to the surgeon, the woman, who was also a nurse, was given radiation and other appropriate therapies; on her own, however, she decided to attend one of Olga Worrall's healing sessions. During the laying on of hands, the nurse reported "the sensation of a big corkscrew turning in my stomach." The tumor, described as the size of a person's head, was still obviously present after the treatment. Yet as time passed the woman became strong enough to return to her job, and within about six months, x-rays showed no trace of the cancerous mass.

Skeptics may argue that the cancer had gone into remission or that the orthodox therapies had brought about the healing, but the nurse and the surgeon felt some other force—transmitted through Olga Worrall—had played a significant role in the woman's cure. More remarkable still, the Worralls sometimes seemed able to bring this healing energy to bear on people who were miles away. This phenomenon was not entirely new in the annals of healing. In the early 1800s, a German nobleman and Catholic healer, with the resounding name of Alexander Leopold Franz Emmerich von Hohenlohe-Waldenburg-Schillingsfürst, was said to have cured faraway patients on at least two occasions

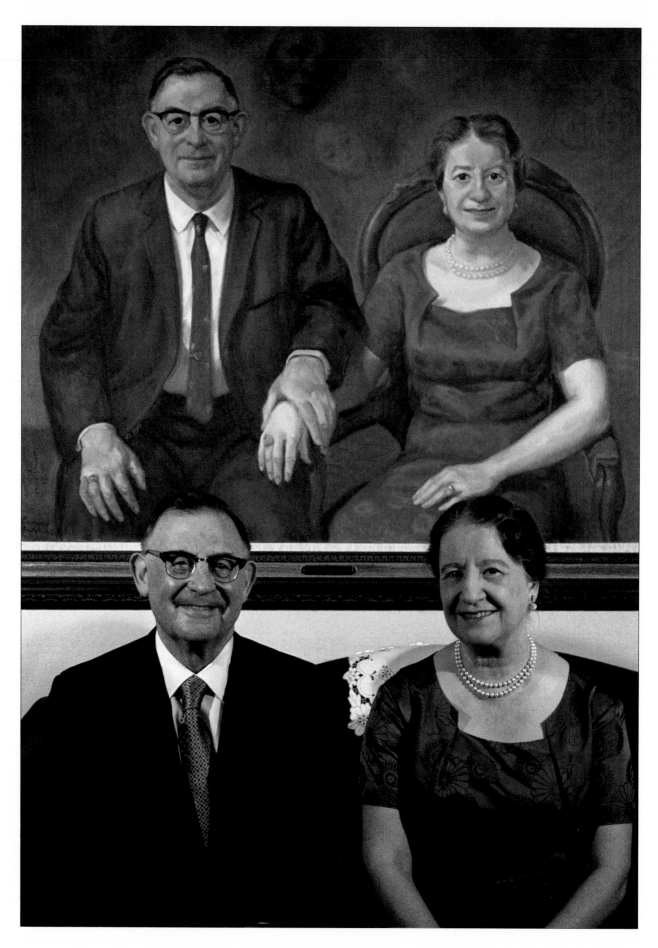

simply by praying for them at his church in Bavaria; one was a novice nun suffering from blood poisoning in Chelmsford, England, the other the paralytic sister of the mayor of Washington, D.C.

Nevertheless, it was a rare gift the Worralls exhibited one day in 1955 when they learned of the predicament faced by a New York City woman named Eleanor Roberts. She had suffered a cerebral aneurysm—a dangerous swelling of a blood vessel in her brain that needed to be repaired by surgery before it ruptured. But surgeons said her temperature was dangerously high, and the operation would have to be delayed until the fever subsided.

The family was in dismay until the woman's brother thought of the Worralls. Telephoning Baltimore, he spoke to Olga, who said that her husband, Ambrose, would be passing through New York that afternoon on his way home from a trip. If someone could meet him at the airport with a photograph of Mrs. Roberts, the Worralls would both pray for her that evening. The contact was made and the prayers said at 9:00 p.m., while Mrs. Roberts lay alone in her room in the New York hospital.

More than thirty years later, Eleanor Roberts said she never forgot the emanations of strength and peace that coursed through her head and body at the moment of prayer that evening. By the next morning, she related, her fever was gone, and the surgeons were able to operate. Subsequently, the Worralls made absent prayer sessions a part of their routine. It was a way to assist, if they could, all the people who called or wrote for help.

As the Worralls seemed to demonstrate with their long-distance treatments, healing need not take place in a formal religious atmosphere. Ruth Carter Stapleton, the sister of former president Jimmy Carter, was a well-known Christian healer who was not ordained or associated with any church. A native of Plains, Georgia, Stapleton traveled all over the United States and abroad, healing with what she considered to be the God-given powers of love, forgiveness, and "prayer through Jesus Christ." To heal the sick, she once explained, "the actual unconditional love of Jesus

has got to be communicated on the unconscious level to the person. Love is the healing agent."

Stapleton's work began in the early 1960s, when her young son Scotty was hit by a car and fell into an apparently fatal coma. At that point, Mrs. Stapleton underwent what she described as a "mystical experience." All anger and anxiety disappeared. She was filled with a feeling of love and joy and peace. She began to sing. That night at the hospital, she sat by her son's bedside and continued to experience what she described as "this terrific internal rejoicing." In the morning, Scotty awoke, fully returned to consciousness. She felt then that "there is something unseen which we can work with to allow miraculous things to happen."

Some years later, in the 1980 book *The New Healers: Healing the Whole Person,* Stapleton recounted how she and two other healers met for a weekend with thirty-five highly skeptical medical doctors. There were question and answer sessions, and "the going was very rough." The doctors brought patients to be treated before the assembly. That went poorly as well. Then a father requested privacy and brought in his son, who had been through five open-heart operations. One of the procedures involved transplanting veins from one of the boy's arms into his chest cavity; as a result, the child was left with one arm shorter than the other. The healers prayed for twenty minutes, at the end of which the father held out his son's arms: They appeared to be the same length. "My God. My God. I can't believe it," cried the father, "He's healed." The father, according to Stapleton, turned out to be one of the most prominent medical doctors at the meeting. The next day, he addressed the assembled group of physicians and healers, she recalled, explaining his son's condition "in scientific, medical terms, and he also described the experience of healing on the previous night. He said he stayed awake all night, and every thirty minutes he measured his son's arms and back to see if he retained the healing."

Many modern-day healers look for help in the spirit world rather than in established religion. Blanche Meyerson, a New York City healer, explains that her energies are

95

sent to her by six "doctors on the other side." If asked, she will name and describe them and tell which are her favorites. "They do the work," she says, "I can't control, or direct it." Her first hints that she had been chosen as a conduit from the spirit world, she explains, came when friends who were psychics relayed messages from the " 'doctors' telling me I should and could treat the sick, that the doctors were ready to work through me." Some time later, she was at a restaurant when one of her dinner companions suddenly toppled over, gasping and turning blue. "I felt myself propelled out of my seat, my right hand leading the way," she recalls. "I reached out. No, it reached out and went straight to his chest." Sparks seemed to fly, she experienced a heavy jolt, and the man was suddenly all right again. "My friend who is psychic told me that he'd had a clot and that the energy dissolved it."

Most often, on instructions from her spirit guides, Meyerson treats patients with a massage-like laying on of hands. Her patients sing her praises—new mothers who had consulted her for help in conceiving, people whose heart conditions are said to have improved, cancer patients whose diseases allegedly went into remission.

Another New York healer, Barbara Ann Brennan, claims her roots are in the ancient universal life forces. She describes her technique as "a laying on of hands that involves rebalancing the Human Energy Field that exists around all of us." That is approximately what Franz Mesmer originally set out to do. But what comes next transcends Mesmer and his disciples in hypnotism.

When she was a young girl growing up in Wisconsin, Brennan had few friends within easy reach. So she spent most of her play hours alone, she recalls, sitting patiently in the woods, waiting for birds and small animals to come up to her. "In those quiet moments in the woods," she explains. "I entered into an expanded state of consciousness in which I was able to perceive things beyond the normal human ranges of experience." She remembers knowing where each small animal was without looking at it. "I could sense its state," she says. "And when I practiced walking

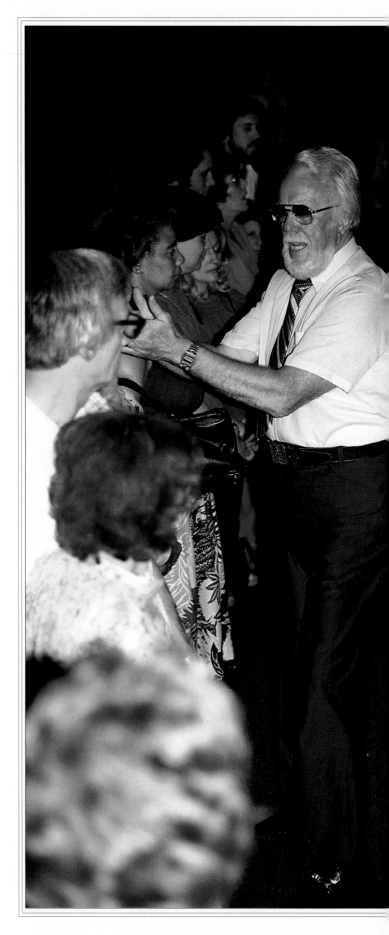

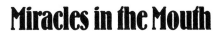

Miracles in the Mouth

No branch of faith healing claims results that strain credulity more than psychic dentistry. While other healers' cures might be explained as psychosomatic reactions, the touch of a dental healer's hand to a believer's cheek allegedly can mend cavities with gold, silver, or porcelain fillings that sometimes materialize before astonished witnesses or even cause new living teeth to sprout in adult jaws.

Believers credit some 25,000 such so-called miracles in the mouth to Willard Fuller, America's foremost dental faith healer. A preacher who says he is only a channel for God's power, Fuller was inspired to try miraculous dental repairs in 1960, after watching evangelist A. C. McKaig, who pioneered the specialty.

Fuller's method is a simple one. He gently strikes the cheeks of those in need and says, "In the name of Jesus, be thou whole." Witnesses who claim to have peered into a mouth to watch the formation of a filling describe it as a small bright spot that expands to fill the whole cavity. One sixty-six-year-old woman, who originally hoped only for a better fit for her dentures, said that within three weeks of Fuller's healing she had cut a new set of thirty-two mature, fully formed teeth.

Fuller's work has never been demonstrated under scientifically controlled conditions. Believers say scientists and medical doctors have witnessed the healings but "most refuse to allow their names to be used." Skeptics cite sleight of hand and patients' self-deception for the seemingly wondrous results. Fuller, an apparently sincere man who does not charge for healing, makes no guarantees, since he believes the healing is inextricably tied to faith. And when he has problems with his own teeth, he goes to a conventional dentist.

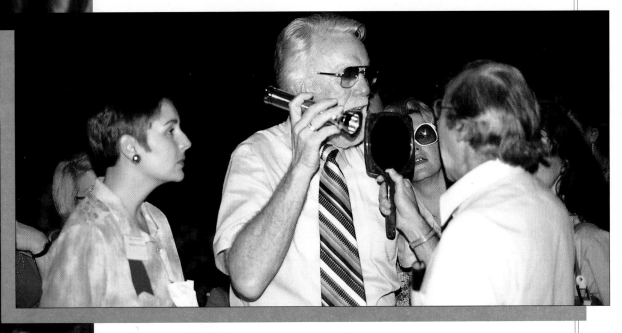

At left, dental faith healer Willard Fuller works his way along a line of the hopeful, supposedly effecting miraculous dentistry by tapping their cheeks with his hands. Later (above), he shines a flashlight into a patient's mouth so the man can see the finished work for himself, while Margaret Fuller, the healer's wife and assistant, looks on.

97

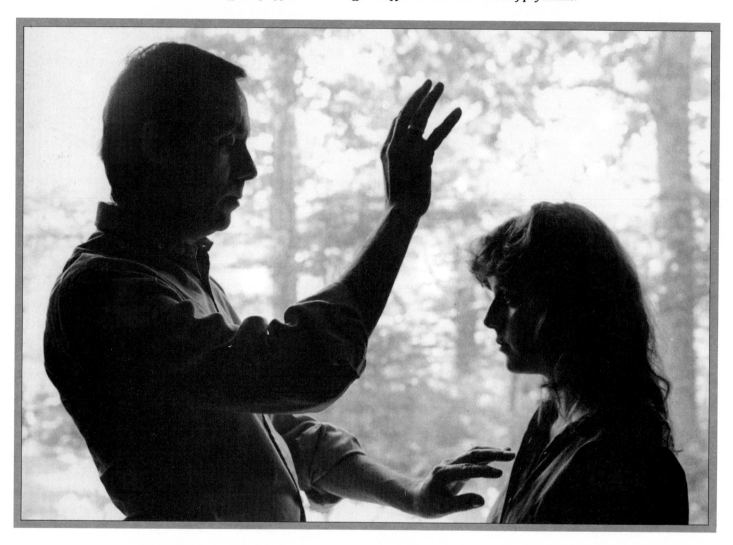

blindfolded in the woods, I would feel the trees long before I could touch them with my hands. I realized that the trees were larger than they appeared to the visible eye." She claims she was learning that trees had energy fields around them, "that everything has an energy field around it that looks somewhat like the light from a candle. Everything was connected by these energy fields. Everything, including me, was living in a sea of energy."

Brennan took a master's degree in atmospheric physics and worked for some years as a NASA researcher before turning to healing full time. She had begun to see colors and shapes around people's heads and remembered her childhood experiences in the woods. It was the beginning, she says, of High Sense Perception (the capitalization is hers), which she describes as the ability to read the energy field that surrounds every person. She claims that by means of meditation, she enters an expanded state of consciousness that enables her to diagram a patient's ills. The colors and shapes she sees correspond to the balance of the field: clear colors and complete shapes for healthy people, muddy colors and malformed shapes for those with infirmities.

Brennan reports that at times she also receives a direct verbal message about the state of a person's energy field. On one occasion, when Brennan was with a woman patient, a voice representing "what appeared to be a higher intelligence than myself" announced, "She has cancer." Brennan then saw a small, black, dented triangular shape in the woman's energy field, at one of her lungs. A CAT scan, Brennan says, confirmed a malignant tumor of that size and shape at that precise spot.

The laying on of her hands, combined with High Sense Perception diagnosis and prescription, Brennan believes, enables her to interact with another person's energy field and rebalance it. She describes a busy day in October 1984. Her first patient, whom she calls Jenny, had miscarried some months before and had been told by her doctor that there were abnormal cells in her uterus where the placenta had been attached. The doctor recommended a hysterectomy, which of course would preclude any further childbearing. During a healing session at that time, Brennan "saw" the abnormal cells in HSP and "heard" what to do about the condition. Jenny was to take a month off, live at the seashore, go on a regime of certain vitamins, follow a specific diet, and meditate for two hours daily. She should then return for further tests that would find her entirely normal. On that day in October 1984, Jenny jubilantly reported that her new tests had in fact been normal, and a year later she gave birth to a fine, healthy baby boy.

Healer Brennan described three other patients she saw on that October day: Howard, whose constant heart pain was responding to a hands-on rebalancing energy transfer; Ed, whose joint problems were traced to an old coccyx injury that responded to an unblocking of the spinal energy flow; and Muriel, whose greatly enlarged thyroid was scheduled for surgery but was so readily reduced by energy healing that surgery proved to be unnecessary. Comments Brennan, "It is as if my life has been guided by some unseen hand that brought me to and led me through each experience in a step-by-step fashion, very much like going to school—the school we call life."

Barbara Ann Brennan is by no means alone today in her belief that she has the power to heal through some form of extrareligious life force. Among modern "hand healers," there are dozens of men and women who claim similar powers—and claim results to show for their belief.

In England, a noted hand healer named Matthew Manning says he discovered at an early age that he possessed psychokinetic powers, that he could move objects around simply by willing them to do so. As an adult, he has supposedly channeled his energies into healing with remarkable effect. A patient is first asked to describe his or her symptoms; Manning then stands behind the person and places his hands on his or her shoulders. His hands begin to move as if of their own volition, seeking out the pain or an organ perhaps related to the disease. All the while, in his mind's eye, Manning, like Brennan, says he is receiving information in color code as to the nature of the disease: red for pain, yellow for infection, black for cancer.

As Manning's hands move over the body, the patient may go into a slight trance. Some patients say they feel heat; it can be mild or so intense as to be almost unbearable, yet there is no actual rise in body temperature. Alternatively, some patients report chills or a sensation of pins and needles running along their limbs or spine. But ordinarily there is no reaction until the patient suddenly exclaims that the pain is receding or that an arthritic limb can be moved for the first time in a long while. The healing sessions last about thirty minutes, and Manning estimates that about two out of every three patients gain relief.

In the Soviet Union—where there is less official antagonism to such supernormal phenomena than in the West, if government research programs are any indication—a onetime Moscow waitress named Dzhuna Davitashvili has won fame by treating patients with a life-giving force called bioenergy. Bioenergy draws on the theories of prana and qi, those animating energies of ancient Eastern belief. According to Davitashvili and other Eastern European healers who employ the technique, bioenergy streams forth from the palms of the hands, unblocking and replenishing the depleted energies of the ill. No less a personage than Leonid Brezhnev, whose slurred speech and halting walk marked him as a very sick man in the winter of 1979, is said to have sought treatment at the healing hands of Davitashvili; by the following spring, the Soviet leader was showing a dramatic improvement. (Although apparently not a permanent cure—he died less than three years later.) And with fame came fortune for the erstwhile waitress, who reportedly has a full calendar of waiting Soviet celebrities, at the equivalent of $275 a session.

In the United States, polarity therapy, a healing practice popular with so-called New Age followers, also uses hands-on techniques supposedly to release energy blockages, but with an interesting variation. Introduced by Austrian physician Randolph Stone in the early 1900s, polarity therapy divides the body into poles of positive and negative energy—the top of the body and right side are positive; the lower extremities and left side are negative. Polarity therapists reportedly heal by a sort of "jumper cable" effect, by transmitting positive and negative charges from their own bodies, or "batteries" (right hand positive, left hand negative), to a patient's body. Depending on the nature of the imbalance, the right hand's positive energy can be used to strengthen the body, while the left hand's negative energy will tend to sedate and relax.

Polarity healers, by means of manipulation and massage, attend to what they recognize as five energy centers—one governing voice, hearing, and throat, another the respiratory and circulatory systems, a third the digestive tract, a fourth the pelvic and glandular centers, and finally, a center controlling the elimination system. The aim of polarity therapy is not to relieve symptoms or cure specific ailments but to realign the body's posture. This, practitioners claim, will maximize the body's preventive and healing powers.

Box That Gives an Orgone Boost

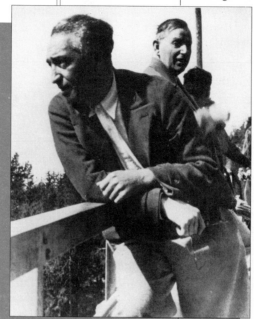

Wilhelm Reich, shown above with his colleague Ola Raknes in the late 1930s, believed an all-encompassing force, orgone energy, determined the weather, as well as human health.

Wilhelm Reich is most widely remembered for inducing followers to sit in refrigerator-size boxes, seeking to cure their ills and improve their sex lives. But the creator of that improbable therapy also promoted some notions that today are regarded as genuine contributions to common-sense healing practices.

Reich, an Austrian-born psychoanalyst, believed that people protect themselves against painful emotions by developing "armor," which eventually manifests itself as chronic muscular tension. "Armoring," Reich said, prevents the release of sexual-emotional energy and often results in mental and physical disorders. Initially, he prescribed a combination of analysis, massage, and breathing exercises to loosen the armor. But in the early 1940s, after moving to Ameri-

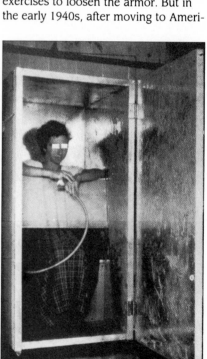

A patient perches on a built-in bench in one of Reich's orgone boxes, ready for the door to be closed for the treatment—thirty minutes or less of just sitting. The tube she holds is intended to funnel orgone energy directly onto afflicted parts of the body.

ca, he became obsessed with what he called orgone energy, a name created by combining the word *orgasm* with the suffix *-one* (as in hormone). He identified orgone not only as sexual energy, but as a cosmic life force pervading the whole universe.

He declared this energy could be collected and applied therapeutically by his orgone energy accumulator, also called the orgone box. Reich said a patient sitting in the accumulator—a cubicle made of layers of wood, steel wool, iron, and other materials, without any moving or electronic parts —could gain relief from many ailments, including impotence and cancer. Federal authorities disapproved: In 1957, he was imprisoned for the interstate distribution of his devices. He died that year at the age of sixty.

Alexander Lowen studied with Reich from 1940 to 1952. Although he rejected the orgone theory, he drew on Reich's work, developing a mind-body therapy he called bioenergetics. According to Lowen, bioenergetics raises the body's energy level, promotes self-expression, and restores the flow of feeling—in other words, loosens the armor. This is done through deep-breathing exercises and movement as well as psychotherapy. Bioenergetic analysis today is practiced and taught in many countries, and the same or similar therapy techniques are widely used by practitioners and clients who may be unaware of the term *bioenergetics* and the name Wilhelm Reich.

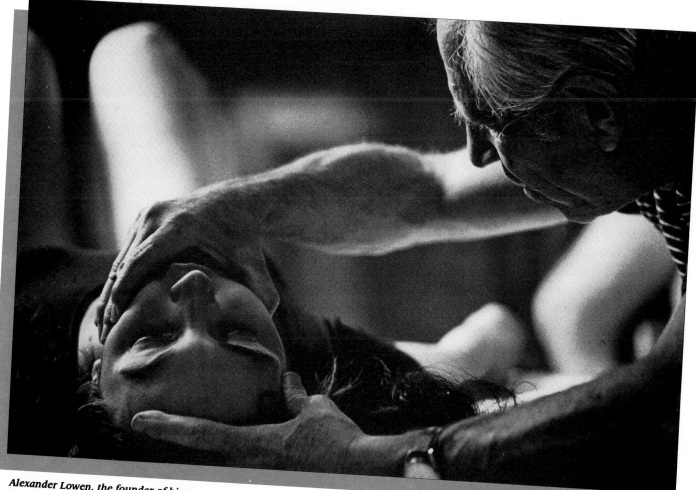

Alexander Lowen, the founder of bioenergetic analysis, helps a client find the proper body alignment for breathing exercises. Increasing energy by maximizing the amount of oxygen intake is a key component of bioenergetics. Lowen maintains that the body's energy processes determine the workings of the mind as well as of the body.

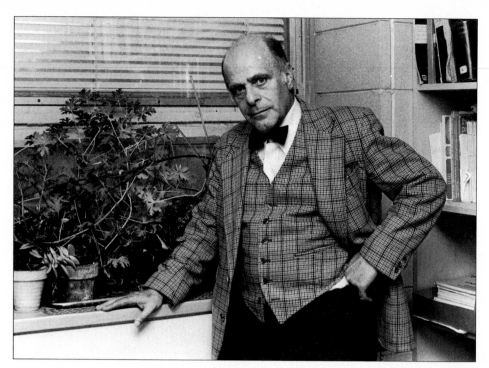

Since the dawn of the Age of Enlightenment and Louis XVI's royal investigation into mesmerism, scientists have been unimpressed by the layers-on of hands and other unorthodox healers. Most authorities have scoffed—when they have exhibited any interest at all. Yet in recent times, a number of researchers have launched serious studies into the phenomena of healing by touch, gesture, and faith.

Most of the scientists looking into such matters have concentrated on the physical energy that seems to emanate from the hands of certain healers. At Montreal's McGill University in the early 1960s, biochemist Bernard Grad undertook a series of laboratory experiments with a well-known hand healer named Oskar Estebany. A one-time Hungarian cavalry colonel, Estebany had enjoyed extraordinary success in ministering to his unit's horses and, in Canada after World War II, had begun to work with humans. In the McGill experiments, however, the subjects were mice, the idea being that animals would have no way of mentally attributing special powers to Estebany and would not adopt a mind-set encouraging a psychosomatic response to his treatments. Thus any healing would be purely and objectively physical.

The mice were induced to develop goiters—chosen because Estebany had a reputation for curing the condition in humans—by means of an iodine-deficient diet. Grad was meticulous in setting up his experiment, establishing three control groups—one treated by Estebany, one that received heat equal to that of Estebany's hands by means of an electrothermal tape, and one that received no heat or handling of any sort. For fifteen minutes twice a day over the course of twenty days, Estebany placed his hands around a wire cage containing nine iodine-deficient mice in individual compartments. At the end of the study, all of the mice were measured for goiter growth. The mice in Estebany's group had significantly less growth than those in the other two groups.

Grad and Estebany went on to test the healer's effect on surgical wounds. And again, the group treated by Estebany exhibited considerably better results than the controls—although critics contended that Estebany's influence was minimal since all the mice healed within the experiment's time frame. Next, Grad had the healer work with barley seeds planted in ordinary peat pots. Estebany did not touch the seeds directly, but treated a beaker of watering solution by holding it for fifteen minutes a day; a control beaker was left untreated. Again he seemed to produce beneficial effects: The seeds watered with the treated solution yielded larger, more abundant plants than the control seeds.

Another researcher—biochemist Justa Smith, a nun at Rosary Hill College in Buffalo, New York—worked with Estebany soon after that to test the hypothesis that a healer's hands exude a magnetic influence on enzyme activity. Estebany was directed to hold a test tube containing an enzyme solution. Since enzymes react to temperature change, the solution was maintained at

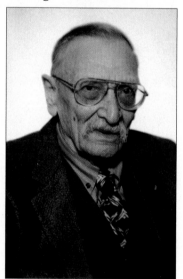

Oskar Estebany, shown here in 1975, was still healing clients at the age of eighty-nine. In his prime, the Hungarian-born healer treated as many as forty people a day, reportedly saving the most challenging cases for the end of the day, at which time, in the words of researcher Bernard Grad, "his energy was really swinging."

a temperature consistent with that of Estebany's body. Periodically, Smith removed a sample from the tube and tested it to see whether the enzyme reaction rate was accelerating over time. It was, and researcher Smith concluded that the effect of Estebany's hands on the enzyme solution was similar to exposing it to a magnetic field. Both stimulated enzyme activity, which she believed might be a key to changing cellular metabolism.

In other experiments, a member of the Soviet Academy of Science reported that Dzhuna Davitashvili had been asked to treat ulcerous skin tissue under laboratory conditions. The academician reported that her healing energy greatly accelerated the "drying out" process by which such ulcers start to heal. The process was completed in scarcely fifteen minutes, wrote the academician, "and five minutes after that, a light pink film appeared, evidencing the formation of skin cells." Similarly, a researcher named Kit Pedler performed an experiment in England with Matthew Manning in which the healer displayed a powerful effect on cell growth. The contents of a flask he was treating exhibited significant biochemical changes over one being held by Pedler and one left entirely alone.

Among the claims of such spiritualist healers as Barbara Ann Brennan and Matthew Manning is that they can discern an energy field emitted by the human body; it appears, they say, as an aura or halo of colors. Some researchers assert this energy field can be captured on film by Kirlian photography, a technique incorporating film and an electrically charged metal plate *(pages 78-79)*. Skeptics are unwilling to consider Kirlian photographs empirical proof in scientific investigations. Yet the medium has created a certain amount of interest. In studies at the University of California at Los Angeles, Thelma Moss reported that Kirlian photographs indicated a far greater level of energy emanation from healers than from ordinary people. What is more, photographs taken of healers' fingers and palms during the act of healing indicated a remarkably stronger aura when the healer was at work than at any other time—Olga Worrall's hands, for example, showed dense orange and red flares of light when she was healing that were not present when she was resting.

Also at UCLA, Valerie Hunt and others have studied the correlation between changes in the very weak natural electrical activity of the body's living tissue and a healer's perception of the body's energy field. Electrodes were attached to a subject's skin in order to record the frequency of low millivoltage signals from the body during a series of deep muscle massages by the technique called rolfing. These signals fed into an oscilloscope, which produced wave forms of different colors on a screen. The Reverend Rosalyn Bruyere of the Healing Light Center in Glendale was in the room during the sessions. She was asked to note the various auras she "saw" and give a running commentary into a tape re-

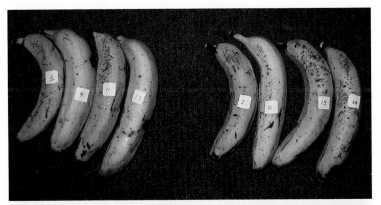

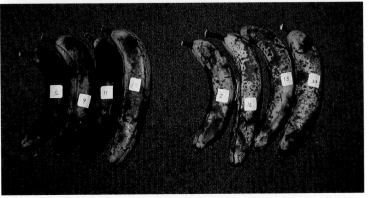

For a 1981 study, Bernard Grad assembled two groups of four bananas, similar in weight and color (top). For seven minutes a day, Grad had healer Georges Ille hold one group in his hands, while a colleague held the other group. On the fourth day, the bananas held by the healer (bottom, left) had become darker than the control group (bottom, right). They were also harder and had lost more weight. Grad concluded that a higher temperature than that normally found in human hands was necessary to produce such effects in bananas.

corder. Bruyere's perceptions were then matched against the electronic signals—and were consistently found to agree with them. When Bruyere reported seeing a blue aura emanating from the subject's thigh as it was being massaged, for instance, the electrode connected to that area relayed a signal that produced a blue wave form on the screen. This seemed to indicate that healers could, in fact, pinpoint and identify the body's various energy emanations.

On the other hand, Julius Weinberger, a consultant physicist for the Radio Corporation of America, has not had great success in capturing x-rays or other evidence of the so-called healing force that practitioners claim to transmit to their ailing subjects. Weinberger began by disbelieving that nonmedical healing "is the result of successfully persuading a capricious deity to set aside the order of the universe." Rather, he felt that such healing "is just as subject to law as are the more commonly encountered healing processes." He thought if he could understand those laws thoroughly, the healing could be repeated at will.

Weinberger used the most sensitive x-ray film obtainable. "We put a bar of lead in front of this package of film," he explained, "and this was fastened on the palms of the healer's hands during the healing treatment." Supposedly, the healer's hands would darken the film but the lead bar would cast a shadow proportionate to its absorption of radiation. He hoped "from the relative density of the covered and unobstructed portions of the film that we would compute the wave length of the radiation." Although the experiment produced no conclusive results, Weinberger was encouraged. "We got more darkening underneath the lead bar than outside of it, as though the lead bar was being excited to emit some form of radiation. In a few other experiments we got faint radiation apparently from an edge of the lead bar, as though this were acting as a dam or obstruction against which the stream of energy momentarily piled up."

In a second test, this time of magnetic properties, Weinberger "took a simple compass to see if two healers could produce any result on that, and they did not." In order to magnify any magnetic effects, Weinberger then added a bar of tool steel at right angles to the compass and asked the healer to put his hands on it. If there was a magnetic force, explained Weinberger, the presence of the bar would multiply the force and the compass needle would change positions as magnetization of the iron was increased. "We tried that," Weinberger said, "and it didn't do anything."

Considering the ambiguous state of scientific inquiry, it is no surprise that the laying on of hands and other supposed supernormal healing methods are regarded with broad skepticism—and not a few charges of outright fraud. Olga Worrall once said that 90 percent of those who loudly tout themselves as faith healers are fakes. As illustration, she liked to recount the story of a dinner party attended by her minister, the Reverend Albert Day. The clergyman noticed that a young woman hired to help serve the meal practically snatched the plates away in her obvious impatience to be finished and gone. As it happened, Mr. Day attended a meeting of a local faith healer after dinner that night. Amid all the shouted amens, who should come limping pitifully down the aisle on crutches but the serving woman. The minister watched with interest as she was touched by the healer—and then hurled away her crutches, exclaiming, "Hallelujah, I am cured!" Catching up with her after the meeting, Mr. Day asked the woman why she had put on such a deceitful show. "Oh, he pays me," she replied. "I come every night and get more money from him than I do in my job."

The record is filled with instances of charlatans exposed. Yet even the most honest and dedicated of healers find themselves pinned in the harsh spotlight of criticism. Among the sharpest of the critics is Dr. William Nolen, a noted Minnesota surgeon. Nolen spent eighteen months examining the literature of psychic healing for cures that he would consider properly documented. He found none.

In his 1974 book, entitled *Healing: A Doctor In Search of a Miracle,* Nolen speaks for many members of the medical profession when he takes aim at magnetic or life force healing. He recounts the case of a magnetic healer he refers to as "Mr. A," whose "inner voices" directed him to cure diseases, including cancer. Mr. A's technique was to "recharge" the patient by placing his hands on the abdomen, that area supposedly being the magnetic center of the body.

In one case, Mr. A claimed credit for curing a cancerous brain tumor in a young woman. In fact, says Nolen, the woman had been operated on by a neurosurgeon prior to visiting Mr. A. The surgeon had found the tumor to be encapsulated, meaning that the malignancy was localized within the covering tissue, a very encouraging sign. The surgeon, says Nolen, removed all the cancer and saved the woman's life; Mr. A deserved no credit whatsoever. Nolen went on to track down twenty-three such cases and discovered not one legitimate cure.

Nolen also takes issue with the faith healers who say, "I don't heal. The Holy Spirit heals through me." That is most convenient, Nolen says. If the patient does not improve, the Holy Spirit gets the blame—or the patient is considered at fault for lacking sufficient faith. Either way, the burden of failure rests elsewhere, rather than with the healer.

Critic Nolen agrees that certain techniques, particularly hypnosis, will heighten a patient's susceptibility to suggestion. And he agrees further that "hypnosis or suggestion will often cure patients, whose symptoms are neither functional nor organic, but, rather, neurotic or hysterical in nature." Such complaints might include a sudden impairment of a sensory function or inexplicable paralysis. A man about to lose his job may wake up one morning blind in one eye, for example, or a woman whose son is arrested for drugs might find she can no longer move her right arm. Nolen calls such phenomena "conversion hysteria" and concedes that healers enjoy some success in those areas. But then so can anyone, he argues, including himself.

The physician relates the case of a patient, Louise, who lost her voice after her husband died in an accident. On examination, her vocal cords were found to be normal, yet four years went by and all she could do was whisper. Then one day Dr. Nolen had to perform gallbladder surgery on her, and afterward he told her a white lie: "Louise, when we operated on you, we had to put a tube into your windpipe to give you the anesthetic. When we did that, I noticed that your vocal cords were stuck together just a bit, so I spread them apart. I'll bet that's why you've had to whisper all these years. By tomorrow I think your voice will be back to normal." The next day, Louise was all smiles and spoke in a normal voice. "It's wonderful, Dr. Nolen," she said. "Spreading those cords did it. Thank you so much."

Some people claim that a crystal swinging over the body's chakras, or energy centers, diagnoses problems: Counterclockwise rotation is believed to signal energy blockage.

Nolen emphasizes, however, that suggestion, faith, or the laying on of kindly hands will not mend a fractured bone or cure a diseased organ. More over, such nonscientific treatment can be extremely dangerous if it masks symptoms and deludes patients so that they fail to consult a qualified medical physician. Nolen recalls the unfortunate case of a woman who was relieved of her excruciating back pain—until her cancerous vertebrae collapsed. "Symptoms—pain, nausea, dizziness—may be purely psychological," says the doctor. "But they may also be warning signals of dangerous organic diseases. When healers treat serious organic diseases, they keep patients away from possibly effective and life-saving help. The healers become killers."

But having offered that judgment, Nolen is quick to say that the medical profession has much to learn in some areas from the healers. Intelligent people seek out alternative therapies because they feel let down by their doctors,

he believes. Cures for widespread cancer, multiple sclerosis, congenital brain disorders are still beyond the powers of orthodox medicine. In such cases, doctors often bluntly tell patients that they cannot help them. But the healers, writes Nolen, "never say, I can't help you." They offer warmth and caring and hope, says Nolen, and "the medical profession can take a lesson in compassion from the healers."

And something else. When all is said and done, nobody can predict with unfailing certainty what any given mind and body are capable of accomplishing. The patient who has faith, whether in a divine higher power or in the benign hands of a charismatic healer, seems to have a better chance of being healed than someone who does not. Nolen has seen too many spontaneous remissions of supposedly terminal cancer to be dogmatic about who will get

California psychologist Richard Heckler guides a client through breathing exercises as part of a healing technique called "bodywork." Heckler's method, which includes talk therapy, touch, and movement, is designed to "better integrate bodies and minds."

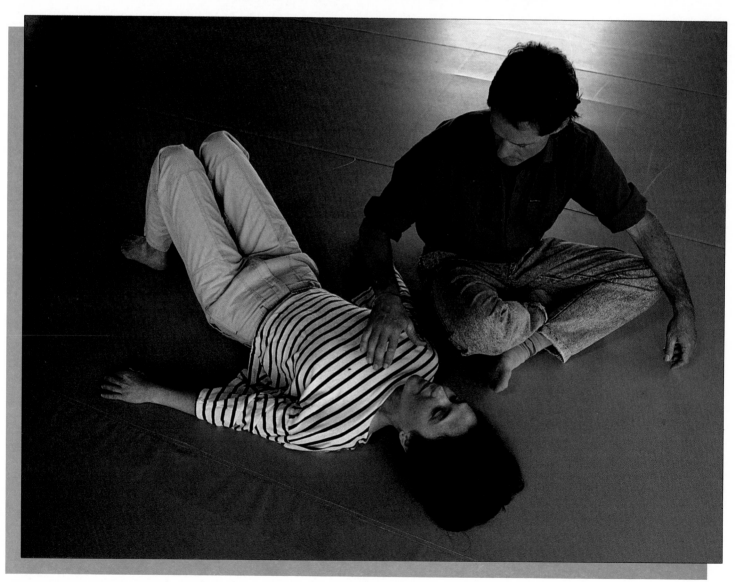

well and who will not. "Show me a doctor who says with certainty that a patient is doomed," he writes, "and I'll show you a damned fool."

That, more or less, was the message of a surprising Supreme Court decision rendered in 1902. One J. H. Kelly had incorporated his American School of Magnetic Healing in Missouri and was peddling through the mails his ability to mentally effect cures over vast distances. For a price, Kelly would set up a time for this telepathic meeting of the minds and allegedly transmit his healing energy; the sufferer had merely to relax and clear away all disturbing thoughts. Kelly was raking in between $1,000 and $1,600 a day when the postmaster general decided to shut him down for mail fraud. Kelly boldly went to court—and won.

Justice Rufus W. Peckham, speaking for the majority, advised the government that it had no right simply to assume that Kelly's mail-order therapy was worthless. "The influence of the mind upon the physical condition of the body is very powerful," wrote Peckham, "and a hopeful mental state goes far, in many cases, not only to alleviate, but even to aid very largely in the cure of an illness from which the body may suffer."

Dolores Krieger would say amen to that. She is a registered nurse with a Ph.D. in the field and holds a position as professor of nursing at New York University. She became interested in healing, particularly in the relationship between the mind and the laying on of hands, because she saw it as a logical extension of her profession. And she saw in healers the same instinct to relieve suffering as that which draws people into nursing.

In 1971, Krieger joined a research team studying what effect, if any, healer Oskar Estebany could have on patients' hemoglobin levels. The results were positive. Under Estebany's laying on of hands, the health-giving red blood cell counts rose. Although skeptical medical professionals have questioned the use of hemoglobin as a variable and cite other methodological problems, Krieger became an enthusiast. She embarked on another experiment—to see whether touch healing was the gift of a very few or whether it was a latent human talent that could be cultivated by anyone.

Little by little, Krieger claims, she mastered the sensitivities of the healer. By her account, she learned to feel different responses when moving her hands over a patient—heat, coolness, tingling. And, she said, she learned to establish such strong communication with patients that she could bring them relief by unblocking their congested energy or infusing them with her own.

There is no great mystery to Dolores Krieger's Therapeutic Touch, as she calls it. "The therapeutic use of hands is a universal human act, a natural human potential, not reserved to a chosen few," according to Krieger. She has personally taught the technique to more than 20,000 people since the 1970s; the majority of those students have been nurses, and among them, only a handful have failed to achieve the touch. She is proud to write that her system is taught in more than eighty U.S. universities and colleges, that it is incorporated into numerous hospital programs, and that it is practiced in thirty-eight foreign countries.

Krieger works strictly within the medical profession and claims no miracle cures, no magical mending of broken spines or clogged hearts. Her touch is notably good in achieving two goals: It provokes a profound feeling of relaxation in the patient, and it is highly effective in relieving pain, both important in assisting the healing process over a wide range of maladies.

But how much of this technique's success involves actual transference of energy and how much can be chalked up to the placebo effect remains to be judged. As with many other alternative therapies, conclusive empirical evidence has not been found for the effectiveness of Therapeutic Touch or other forms of laying on of hands, despite the encouraging indications revealed by the studies of Oskar Estebany. However, that does not mean these therapies do not excite interest or that there is not still a vast amount of research to be done. As Krieger so aptly observes, "The deeper we study the dynamics of healing, the more one is impressed by how little we really know about the healing act."

A Gallery of Unproved Therapies

Can a quartz crystal cure arthritis? Do certain colors have healing powers? Will inhaling an aromatic herb or flower relieve stress—or, better yet, cure the common cold? Across America and around the world, there are thousands of people—practitioners and devotees of alternative medicine—who swear that all these things are indeed possible.

Each of the four unorthodox therapies described below and on the following six pages employs natural tools: colors, crystals, essential oils, and flower essences. They also are patterned after holistic principles. That is, their practitioners, who usually style themselves as healers or therapists, seek to understand the physical makeup as well as the psychological makeup of their clients. Typically, they hold that many ailments are the result of imbalances in the body's energy or emotional makeup, which they attempt to treat—often in conjunction with more traditional medical care.

Many say they have found these alternative therapies to be helpful. But there is little or no scientific evidence to bolster their assertions, and anyone with symptoms of an actual illness should consult a qualified medical physician.

A Colorful Cure for the Blues

In the 1930s, Indian-born Dinshah Ghadiali advertised that he could cure everything from cancer to lumbago merely by exposing patients to intense colored light. Not surprisingly, he was branded a charlatan by the American Medical Association and forced out of business by the Food and Drug Administration.

But his faith in the healing properties of color was not without precedent. Ancient Egyptians treated patients with colored light. Indian philosophers held that color was as vital to one's well-being as air.

A growing number of so-called color therapists claim that a wide range of dis-

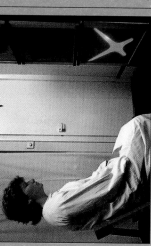

Bathed in an orange light, this patient hopes to benefit from the supposedly curative effects of color therapy.

orders can be cured by colored light and the right colors in food, clothing, and décor. Many believe the seven colors of the spectrum correspond to the seven chakras, or energy centers, said to run along the spine. Although some color therapy notions are widely accepted—hospitals, for instance, decorate rooms in colors thought to be soothing and thus therapeutic—critics say it is dangerous to assert that patients can be cured just by correcting a "color imbalance." But color therapists stand by their claims and ascribe distinct healing powers to each of the spectrum's colors, as shown below.

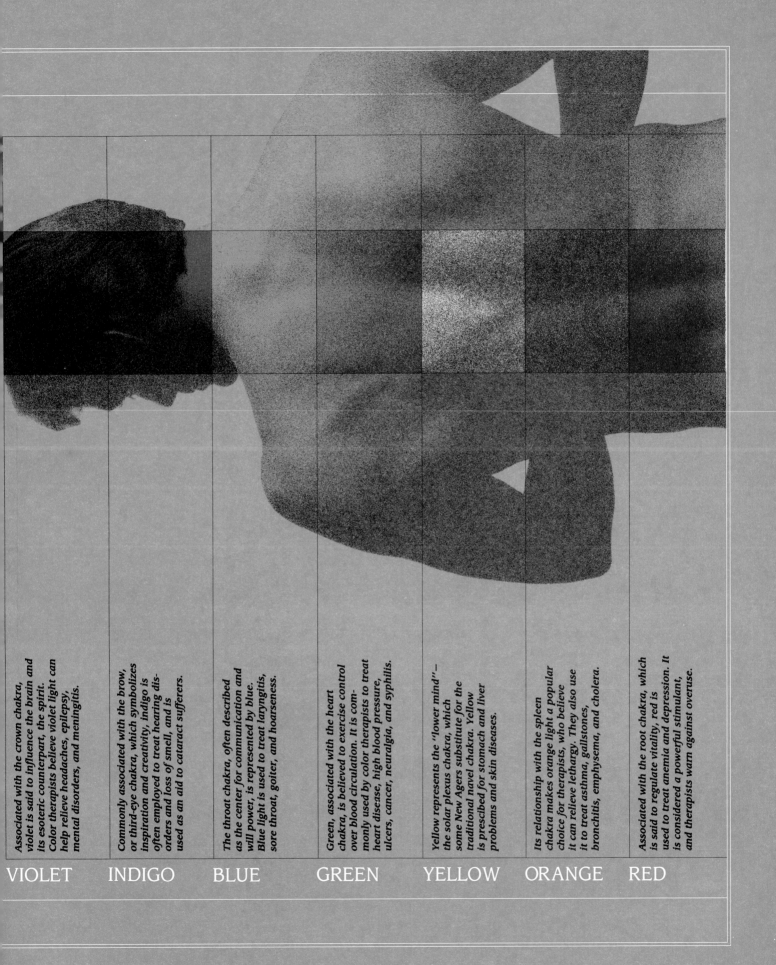

Associated with the crown chakra, violet is said to influence the brain and its esoteric counterpart, the spirit. Color therapists believe violet light can help relieve headaches, epilepsy, mental disorders, and meningitis.

Commonly associated with the brow, or third-eye chakra, which symbolizes inspiration and creativity, indigo is often employed to treat hearing disorders and loss of smell, and is used as an aid to cataract sufferers.

The throat chakra, often described as the center for communication and will power, is represented by blue. Blue light is used to treat laryngitis, sore throat, goiter, and hoarseness.

Green, associated with the heart chakra, is believed to exercise control over blood circulation. It is commonly used by color therapists to treat heart disease, high blood pressure, ulcers, cancer, neuralgia, and syphilis.

Yellow represents the "lower mind"— the solar plexus chakra, which some New Agers substitute for the traditional navel chakra. Yellow is prescibed for stomach and liver problems and skin diseases.

Its relationship with the spleen chakra makes orange light a popular choice for therapists, who believe it can relieve lethargy. They also use it to treat asthma, gallstones, bronchitis, emphysema, and cholera.

Associated with the root chakra, which is said to regulate vitality, red is used to treat anemia and depression. It is considered a powerful stimulant, and therapists warn against overuse.

VIOLET   INDIGO   BLUE   GREEN   YELLOW   ORANGE   RED

Crystal Consciousness

In New Mexico, a woman places crystals on the chest of a leukemia sufferer in order to cure him. A New York businessman never leaves home without taking a small crystal; he claims it helps him concentrate. Another believer uses a crystal as a deodorant, rubbing it under his arms.

The phenomenon that some have dubbed "crystal consciousness" began spreading across the U.S. in the mid-1980s. Devotees attribute paranormal healing and restorative powers to gemstones such as clear quartz crystal, amazonite, amethyst, and aventurine. There is no scientific evidence to support their claims, but some crystal therapists allege that they have relieved ailments such as bursitis, Parkinson's disease, and even blindness by exposing clients to crystals. Faith in the power of crystals is not

new. The ancient Greeks used the stones to cauterize wounds, and many maintain that crystal jewelry was originally worn to ward off disease. Some believers claim that the Maya and Sumerians used the stones for healing and contend that the Egyptian pyramids were once capped with quartz intended to channel cosmic forces.

"Crystals are tools, not an end in themselves," says Katrina Raphaell, founder of the Crystal Academy of Advanced Healing Arts in Taos, New Mexico. Crystals, she explains, are used to tap an individual's own inner healing power. Raphaell selected the crystals shown below and described their alleged properties. Some are said to apply to particular chakras, or energy centers. Caution: Anyone suffering from any of these illnesses should seek a qualified medical doctor's help.

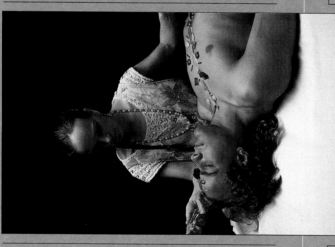

Crystal healer Katrina Raphaell applies a variety of crystals to a client. An azurite nodule placed between the eyebrows is intended to "unblock the unconscious."

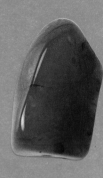

Green aventurine, placed atop the solar plexus chakra, allegedly connects the upper, mental body with the lower, physical one, frees blocked energy, and allows deep, healing breathing.

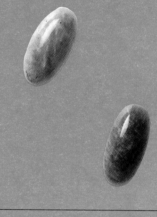

Crystal therapists say the red-orange agate carnelian serves as an energizer and blood purifier and helps absent-minded or unfocused people. When placed atop the spleen chakra, carnelian is believed to stimulate creative expression.

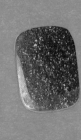

When placed atop the throat chakra, amazonite is thought to help a person talk about repressed feelings. It supposedly links the mind and the heart, since it is used on the chakra positioned between the two.

The commonest of all crystals, the clear quartz is usually placed on the top of the head, at the crown chakra, and is reputed to stimulate the light-sensitive pineal gland and activate higher consciousness.

The amethyst crystal, placed over the third-eye chakra, is considered the principal meditation stone. The purple crystal purportedly calms both the conscious and subconscious mind and is commonly held or worn while meditating.

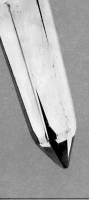
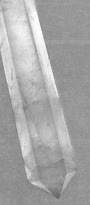
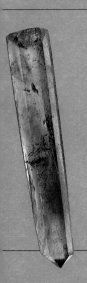

At the heart chakra, rose quartz is said to aid in achieving self-love and inner peace, thought to be the first step in the healing process. Crystal therapists advise clients to carry or wear rose quartz to help gain harmony with themselves.

One of the most brilliant of all the dark stones, smoky quartz purportedly transforms the body's spiritual energy into healing power when placed over the root chakra. Therapists advise that smoky quartz should be used with care.

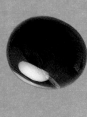
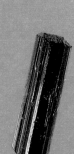

Black tourmaline is said to deflect negative energies instead of absorbing them. Its parallel striations supposedly help channel the healing effects of higher frequency spiritual energy. Believers also carry the stone when psychic protection is needed.

Bicolored watermelon tourmaline is said to be the best available healer of the heart chakra. The green ray allegedly treats the emotional wounds the heart has stored, while the pink allegedly inspires the flow of love.

Believers in crystals think azurite's deep indigo blue helps penetrate subconscious blockages. Because of its supposed power, advocates say it should be used only when a person is psychologically ready, lest it produce fearful reactions in one unprepared for the insight and clarity of vision it brings.

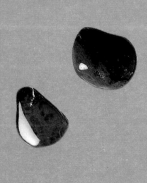
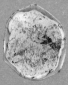

Considered to be an important healing stone, bloodstone is said to purify the blood and is sometimes used in detoxification, when it is placed over the liver or kidneys.

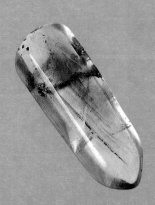

The stone commonly associated with creativity, fluorite is said to balance the intuitive and intellectual aspects of the mind. Described as a third-eye stone, it is intended to help the mind maintain a meditative space at all times.

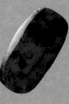

Dense and opaque, sugilite is often used by crystal healers on the lymph nodes of AIDS sufferers and placed over the diseased areas of cancer victims. It is thought to channel spiritual healing from the mind into the body.

Citrine is recommended for situations in which one needs to feel confident and secure. It is purported to help identify personal powers and harness them to achieve goals.

Gem silica, its powers heightened by flecks of malachite, is often used to treat feminine disorders such as menstrual discomfort and may be held while giving birth. It is also said to ease the pain of sorrow and the strain of anger. Men are advised to use the stone to achieve greater vulnerability and sensitivity.

Aroma Therapy: Scents or Nonsense?

In the 1920s, when French chemist René Maurice Gattefossé badly burned his hand in a laboratory experiment, he plunged it into a nearby jar of lavender oil. Although he was not surprised that the oil numbed the pain, Gattefossé was amazed that it also appeared to hasten healing.

The chemist, now known as the father of aroma therapy, began investigating the therapeutic properties of essential oils, so called because they embody the essence—the volatile distillation of odor, taste, and other qualities—of plants such as basil, jasmine, sage, and lavender. His research opened the way for today's self-described healers who claim to cure colds, menstrual cramps, skin diseases,

and a laundry list of other ailments.

Like other unorthodox healing methods, aroma therapy (or *aromatherapy*, as its adherents like to spell it) claims historical antecedents. As early as the fifteenth century BC, aromatics were in wide use as medicines. The Bible makes reference to healing with aromatic oils. And in the Middle Ages, aromatic resins were burned to purify the air during the Great Plague.

Today's aroma therapists say that the oils of various plants can be effective when taken internally, inhaled, or applied externally. And although physicians reject most of the claims made for the therapeutic powers of aromatic oils, even skeptics acknowledge the restorative benefits of

the substances when used in a relaxing rubdown or bath.

The information below is from a chart by British aroma therapist Robert B. Tisserand. The table is divided into four groups by which aroma therapists classify the oils: regulators, stimulants, sedatives, and euphorics. The terms may bear no relation to the meanings of the same words in conventional, scientific medicine. Tisserand advises that "anyone who is seriously ill should consult a qualified medical practitioner." In fact, most of the illnesses below are serious by definition, and caution dictates that anyone with such symptoms should see a medical doctor immediately.

STIMULANTS

Essential Oil	Problems It Is Used For	Methods of Use
PEPPERMINT *Mentha piperita*	Mental fatigue, concentration or memory difficulties, indigestion, nausea, flatulence, muscular and joint aches and pains	Inhalation, bath, vaporization, medicine, massage
EUCALYPTUS *Eucalyptus globulus*	Colds, influenza, bronchitis, arthritis, muscular pain, infections, immune deficiency	Inhalation, massage, vaporization
JUNIPER *Juniperus communis*	Cystitis, urinary infections, arthritis, gout, menstrual cramps, light menstrual flow	Medicine, massage
ROSEMARY *Rosmarinus officinalis*	Mental fatigue, poor memory, arthritis, muscular aches, immune deficiency	Inhalation, bath, vaporization, massage
TEA-TREE *Melaeuca altemifolia*	Burns, insect bites and stings, mouth ulcers, athlete's foot, ringworm, nailbed infections, cystitis, thrush	Frequently repeated applications to affected areas, medicine, massage

REGULATORS

Essential Oil	Problems It Is Used For	Methods of Use
BERGAMOT *Citrus bergamia*	Anxiety, depression, eczema, dermatitis	Massage, bath, vaporization
FRANKINCENSE *Boswellia thurifera*	Fears, nightmares, premature aging, rheumatoid arthritis	Massage, bath, vaporization
GERANIUM *Pelargonium graveolens*	Mood swings, menopausal problems, stomach ulcers, diarrhea	Massage, bath, perfume, medicine
ROSE ABSOLUTE *Rosa centifolia*	Anxiety, emotional trauma, irregular menstruation, impatience, confusion	Massage, bath, perfume
ROSEWOOD *Aniba rosaeodora*	Anxiety, insomnia, mood swings, menstrual cramps, irregularity	Massage, bath, perfume

EUPHORICS

CLARY SAGE *Salvia sclarea*	Depression, menstrual cramps, PMS, throat infections, laryngitis	Massage, bath, perfume, vaporization, gargle
GRAPEFRUIT *Citrus paradisi*	Depression, resentment, gallstones, urinary stones, arterial deposits	Massage, bath, perfume, vaporization, medicine
JASMINE *Jasminum officinale*	Depression, lack of confidence, impotence, frigidity, introversion, emotional coldness	Massage, bath, perfume, vaporization
ROSE OTTO *Rosa damascena*	Depression, grief, hangover, infertility in women	Massage, bath, perfume, compresses
YLANG-YLANG *Cananga odorata*	Depression, anger, impotence, frigidity, hypertension, palpitations	Massage, bath, perfume, vaporization, inhalation

SEDATIVES

CHAMOMILE *Anthemis nobilis*	Anger, irritability, menstrual cramps, heavy menstrual flow, menopausal problems	Massage, inhalation, bath
LAVENDER *Lavandula angustifolia*	Anxiety, insomnia, burns, insect bites and stings, eczema, dermatitis	Massage, bath, inhalation, vaporization, perfume, frequent applications to affected areas
MARJORAM *Origanum marjorana*	Anxiety, stress, hypertension, insomnia, asthma, panic attack	Massage, bath, inhalation
ORANGE BLOSSOM *Citrus aurantium*	Anxiety, stress, palpitations, insomnia, premature aging, immune deficiency	Massage, inhalation, bath, vaporization, perfume
SANDALWOOD *Santalum album*	Stress, fear, insecurity, cystitis, urinary infections, throat infections, laryngitis	Massage, bath, vaporization, medicine, gargle

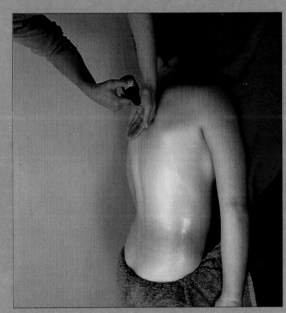

Massage is just one of the methods aroma therapists use to treat clients with essential oils; here, a therapist prepares to apply an oil reputed to have relaxing attributes.

Dr. Bach's Flower Power

In the early 1930s, a renowned British physician, Dr. Edward Bach, noted that many illnesses seemed directly related to the patient's troubled mental state. Believing that traditional medicine neglected the emotions, Bach abandoned his lucrative practice and began to search for a method to "treat the patient and not his disease."

Over the next several years, he formulated what have come to be known as the Bach Flower Remedies, thirty-eight flower-based formulas purported to cure a wide range of emotional problems, including fear, uncertainty, and loneliness. The "remedies" are listed below with the problems to which Bach addressed them.

To prepare his Flower Remedies, Bach ignored his scientific background and relied on intuition. He claimed he could discern the healing properties of a flower merely by placing his hand over its petals. The elixirs, now sold around the world,

are dilute forms of flower and plant extracts in a mix that is 40 percent alcohol, which should be noted by any would-be user sensitive to it. They are still produced only at the Wallingford, Oxfordshire, house where Bach first made them from locally grown flowers.

Supporters credit the nostrums with curing everything from shyness to despondency, and the U.S. Food and Drug Administration has approved them as homeopathic preparations for sale to the general public. But there is no scientific proof of their efficacy, and some of the emotional states they purport to treat warrant consultation with a medical doctor or other qualified counselor.

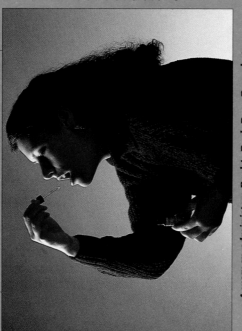

A woman administers Bach's Rock Rose Remedy to herself by placing it under her tongue with an eyedropper. The nostrums can also be swallowed with water.

FEAR

Remedy	Problems It Is Used For	Purported Positive Results
ROCK ROSE *Helianthemum mmularium*	Extreme fear, terror, panic	Heroic bravery, selflessness
MIMULUS *Mimulus guttatus*	Shyness, timidity, known fears	Courage to face all worrying situations without fear
CHERRY PLUM *Prunus cerasifera*	Collapse of mental control, vicious temper, fear of doing harm to self and others	Calm, quiet courage with control over extreme mental pressures
ASPEN *Populus tremula*	Apprehension, foreboding, unknown and vague fears	Fearlessness, faith to face experience and adventure
RED CHESTNUT *Aesculus carnea*	Exaggerated fears for others (especially loved ones), anticipating the "worst"	Genuine concern—but without irrationality

OVERCARE FOR OTHERS' WELFARE

Remedy	Problems It Is Used For	Purported Positive Results
CHICORY *Cichorium intybus*	Possessiveness, demanding respect and obedience, selfishness	Selflessness in care and concern for others
VERVAIN *Verbena officinalis*	Overenthusiasm, fanaticism, nervousness, rage at injustices	Calmness and sureness of mind, control of self, open-mindedness
VINE *Vitis vinifera*	Domination, inflexibility, ambition, strength, tyranny, autocracy	Wisdom, understanding, leadership with great strength, guidance, and help for others
BEECH *Fagus sylvatica*	Intolerance, criticism, arrogance, judgmental tendencies	Tolerance
ROCK WATER (water from well or spring known to have healing power)	Self-denial, rigidity, tightness, self-repression, tendency to set an example, self-righteousness	Idealism with flexible mind, ability to enjoy experiences in life, relaxation

DESPONDENCY AND DESPAIR

Remedy	Negative state	Positive state
LARCH *Larix decidua*	Lack of confidence—anticipation and fear of failure, unwillingness to try, feeling inferior	Perseverance in projects, willingness to try, faith in own ability
PINE *Pinus sylvestris*	Guilt, self-reproach, over-conscientiousness, feelings of unworthiness, taking blame for others' mistakes	Balanced sense of responsibility, refusal to dwell on mistakes made
ELM *Ulmus procera*	Feeling temporarily overwhelmed by responsibility, though normally very capable	Powerful ability to take responsibility, confidence, self-assurance
SWEET CHESTNUT *Castanea sativa*	Extreme anguish, desolation, reaching limit of endurance (nonsuicidal)	Faith that the anguish is a necessary experience but will soon dissipate
STAR OF BETHLEHEM *Ornithogalum umbellatum*	Reactions to fright, serious news, great sorrow, trauma	Body and mind clear of the tensions and residues of trauma
WILLOW *Salix vitellina*	Resentment, bitterness, "it's not fair," "poor me"	Great optimism, less embitterment with life
OAK *Quercus robur*	Inability to struggle bravely against illness and/or adversity though normally strong and courageous	Brave "fighter" without loss of hope, stability, courage
CRAB APPLE *Malus pumilia*	Feeling unclean (in mind or body), self-dislike/disgust	Broadmindedness, genuine self-satisfaction

UNCERTAINTY

Remedy	Negative state	Positive state
CERATO *Ceratostigma willmottiana*	Doubting own judgment, seeking confirmation and advice before acting, acting misguidedly	Quiet assurance, ability to choose correct action, intuition
SCLERANTHUS *Scleranthus annuus*	Uncertainty, indecision (between two choices), vacillation, fluctuating moods	Calmness, determination, poise, balance, quickness in deciding and taking action
GENTIAN *Gentiana amarella*	Despondence, easy discouragement, dejection from known cause	Optimism and perseverance, strength in face of setbacks
GORSE *Ulex europaeus*	Extreme hopelessness, despair, pessimism, negativity, "oh, what's the use"	Positive faith and hope, certainty in overcoming difficulties
HORNBEAM *Carpinus betulus*	Procrastination, "Monday morning feeling" (but usually finishes tasks once they are started)	Sureness in own ability and strength to face problems and "get up and go"
WILD OAT *Bromus ramosus*	Lack of fulfillment, ambition with no determined path, "fish out of water"	Definite ambitions and knowledge of what to do in life

LACK OF INTEREST

Remedy	Negative state	Positive state
CLEMATIS *Clematis vitalba*	Daydreaming, indifference, inattention, escapism	Lively interest in things that are inspired, artistic or down to earth
HONEYSUCKLE *Lonicera caprifolium*	Nostalgia—living in the past, reflecting on past pleasures and glories, homesickness	Retaining wisdom of past while letting go of the experience
WILD ROSE *Rosa canina*	Resignation, apathy, drifting with no ambition	Lively interest in all things, vitality
OLIVE *Olea europaea*	Complete exhaustion, loss of energy, feeling that daily work is a chore	Peace of mind, not drained or overcome by pressures
WHITE CHESTNUT *Aesculus hippocastanum*	Preoccupation with persistent and unwanted worrying thoughts, mental arguments	Quiet and calm mind, undisturbed by outside influences
MUSTARD *Sinapis arvensis*	Deep gloom, melancholia, "dark cloud" coming and going at intervals for no known reason	Unshakable inner serenity, constant stability and joy
CHESTNUT BUD *Aesculus hippocastanum*	Slowness in learning life's lessons, repetition of mistakes	Keen observation of all events, learning from experience

LONELINESS

Remedy	Negative state	Positive state
WATER VIOLET *Hottonia palustris*	Pride, reserve, acting superior or aloof, independence	Gentleness and tranquillity, poise, dignity, grace, sympathy, wisdom
IMPATIENS *Impatiens glandulifera*	Impatience (especially with slow people), hastiness, independence, quickness in thought and action	Understanding and tolerance
HEATHER *Calluna vulgaris*	Overconcern with self, boring overtalkativeness, poor listening, hatred of being alone	Selflessness, helpfulness, control of talking

OVERSENSITIVITY

Remedy	Negative state	Positive state
AGRIMONY *Agrimonia eupatoria*	Inner torture hidden behind a facade of cheerfulness, hiding worries from others	Laughing at one's worries, genuine optimism, sense of humor without pretense
CENTAURY *Centaurium umbellatum*	Weak will, subservience, exaggerated anxiety to please, "doormat" tendency, inability to say no	Quietness, wisdom, serving, knowing when to give or not, maintaining individuality
WALNUT *Juglans regia*	Difficulty in transition or change, wavering before powerful influences	Constancy and determination, faith in personal beliefs, ability to adjust
HOLLY *Ilex aquifolium*	Lack of love for others, envy, jealousy, hatred, suspicion	Generosity, affection, tolerance, happiness whatever the external circumstances

CHAPTER 4

The Mind as Physician

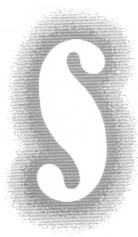ome years ago, a young American East Coast boy was found to have terminal cancer; a malignant tumor had invaded his brain. The doctor told the boy's parents that nothing further could be done; the child would soon die. The parents refused to accept that verdict and took their son to Rochester, Minnesota, to the biofeedback center of the Mayo Clinic, an institution noted for its willingness to consider innovative approaches to medicine. There, a member of the staff discussed with the boy the idea that his mind might be able to influence his disease, that he might be able to help himself by visualizing his cancer and finding ways to combat it.

The boy was reluctant to even try it at first. But he was a vigorous, imaginative youngster, and he finally decided to invent his own mind's-eye video game—with rocket ships zooming vividly around his head, firing their powerful guns at the tumor, which he imagined as "big, dumb and gray." Back home, the child concentrated on his game and steadily blasted away at the invader. One day, after a few months had gone by, he said to his father, "I just took a trip through my head in a rocket ship, and I can't find the cancer anymore."

His parents did not put much stock in that, and when the boy pleaded for another x-ray examination, his doctor advised that it would be a waste of money. But since the boy felt well enough, he returned to school—where he promptly took a tumble on the playground. When the doctor speculated that the tumor had caused the boy's fall, the family asked for a CAT scan, a type of three-dimensional x-ray.

The CAT scan revealed that the tumor was no longer there. It had disappeared without a trace.

This is perhaps the best known and most dramatic of the hundreds of similar reports related regularly in the literature of alternative medicine. Others include the story of how a nurse with cancer gamely and successfully refused to die, just to show her doom-saying doctor—"that S.O.B.," as she called him. How a man with throat cancer adopted a positive attitude toward his radiation treatment—and not only beat the cancer, but cured his crippling arthritis and a twenty-year case of impotence as well. How a frail woman defeated a heart attack, a bleeding ulcer, grief over the death of her husband, and cancer of the breast and chest wall because she remembered her mother's always telling her: "You're scrawny, but whatever happens, you'll always get over it. You'll live to be 93, and then they'll have to run you over with a steamroller."

And consider the experience of the well-known writer and editor Norman Cousins. After he published an account of his remarkable recovery from ankylosing spondylitis (a disease of the body's connective tissue), which he credited in large part to positive thinking and a good doctor-patient relationship, Cousins received a flood of mail from physicians around the world. Some of the letter writers were skeptical. But many doctors supported his conclusions about the mind's ability to heal the body and applauded the idea of forging a partnership between patient and physician in the search for a cure. These doctors, Cousins wrote later, "reflected the view that no medication they could give their patients was as potent as the state of mind that a patient brings to his or her own illness. In this sense, they said, the most valuable service a physician can provide to a pa-tient is helping him to maximize his own recuperative and healing potentialities."

The idea that there is a mental element to healing has gained acceptance within the medical establishment in recent years. Many physicians who once discounted the mind's ability to influence healing are now reconsidering, in light of new scientific evidence. Researchers are probing a variety of phenomena—from the curative value of inert "sugar pills" to how patients can slow their heartbeat simply by will power. Indeed, a new discipline known as psychoneuroimmunology has emerged to study the ties between the psyche and the immune system. All this has led some physicians and medical institutions toward a more holistic approach, to treating the mind and body as a unit rather than as two distinct entities. Inherent in this holistic philosophy is the belief that patients must be active participants in the treatment of their illnesses.

Some contend that holism is nothing new, that medicine has understood the interdependence of mind and body since the days of Hippocrates. They cite Socrates, who said, "There is no illness of the body apart from the mind," and say that for many years physicians have been treating the whole person: Patients with coronary heart disease may be given a number of medications, but they will also be advised to lose weight, quit smoking, exercise regularly, and reduce their mental stress levels.

Some critics argue that the holistic movement goes far beyond that sensible advice and descends into the dark world of occultism. In a 1983 paper entitled "Engineers, Cranks, Physicians, Magicians," which appeared in the *New England Journal of Medicine,* two respected professors of philosophy, Douglas Stalker and Clark Glymour, wrote scathingly of holistic medicine. It is, they conclude, "a pabulum of common sense and nonsense offered by cranks and quacks and failed pedants who share an attachment to magic and an animosity toward reason."

The naysayers trace this "alternative," or "irregular," medicine, as they sometimes call it, back to a nineteenth-century revolt against certain standard medical practices of the day, among them such dubious therapies as bleeding, purging, and blistering. In addition to censuring those cruel practices, however, the irregulars proceeded to devise new therapies based on a sort of faulty empiricism that held, in effect, that if something seems to work once, it must work all the time. The critics offer as a classic of its kind the case of German businessman Carl Baunscheidt, whose rheumatic hand was bitten by gnats one afternoon in 1848. When his rheumatic ache eased just after the gnat attack, Herr Baunscheidt was convinced that he had found nature's own cure in the pesky insects. He thereupon constructed his "Great Resuscitator," a sort of mechanized gnat, with two-inch-long needles to puncture the patient's skin and thereby allow poisonous, pain-causing matter to escape the body.

As the century progressed, nature-reliant medicine, especially homeopathy *(pages 120-121)* won much favor, and practitioners devised lengthy lists of observable symptoms to which they matched lists of remedies. In *The Homeopathist, or Domestic Physician,* a Philadelphia medical doc-

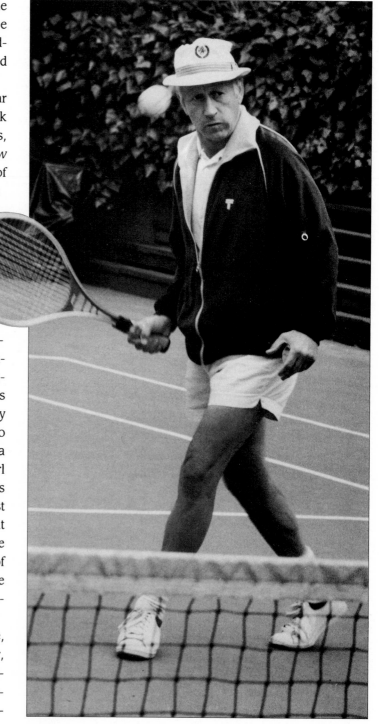

Editor Norman Cousins plays a vigorous game of tennis fifteen years after he battled a painful degenerative disease by reading humorous prose and watching television comedies. He wrote: "I made the joyous discovery that 10 minutes of genuine belly laughter had an anesthetic effect and would give me at least two hours of pain free sleep."

tor named Constantine Hering offered two large volumes of symptoms and cures; the books came with a "domestic kit" of forty broad-spectrum home remedies identified by number. Many of the nostrums were intended for headaches: Remedy number one was appropriate if the head felt "as if the brains were shattered, crushed, burst"; number three, if the ache was accompanied by a "red and bloated" face; number thirteen, if joined by a sudden dislike of coffee; number seventeen, when the headache afflicted "stubborn, unruly children, fond of dainties."

There were various other alternative approaches. Hydropathy, or water cure, enjoyed numerous adherents; spas proliferated, and many of them remain popular to this day. Hydropathy's offshoot, hygeio-therapy, regarded hygiene as next to godliness and prescribed cleanliness, diet, exercise, and fresh air—in addition to the waters—as the sure answer to virtually all maladies.

The most severe of the critics regard such eccentric ideas as the intellectual forerunners of today's medical holism, and they charge holists with practicing the same sort of simplistic and spurious pseudoscience. And yet there is much about holistic medicine, even from its earliest beginnings, that cannot be laughed away. Most of the evidence may be anecdotal but is compelling nonetheless.

Among the first to preach unorthodox medical techniques involving the mind over the body was a sixteenth-century Swiss alchemist with the formidable name of Theophrastus Bombast von Hohenheim—or Paracelsus, as he was commonly known. One of Paracelsus's patients was Johann Froben, a well-known scholar and printer and friend to many influential people, including the great Dutch theologian and humanist Erasmus. In 1527, the story goes, Froben lay abed in Basel, Switzerland, critically ill with an infected leg. Eight doctors had come and gone, and all eight had declared that the leg must be amputated to save Froben's life. Froben was deeply distressed; he loved to hike in the mountains around Basel. How could he continue this pleasure with only one leg?

Froben had heard of Paracelsus, who was then living in Strasbourg, and of his success at curing patients "from within"—without resorting to surgery. He sent the physician a note by special messenger: Would the doctor come and minister to him?

Paracelsus agreed at once and set out on horseback for the seventy-mile journey. Two days later, he was ushered into Froben's sickroom, where he found his patient in great pain. After examining the leg, Paracelsus offered his diagnosis: The leg was in grave danger, but it could be saved if Froben would cooperate totally in the treatment. That would mean undergoing a cure for the entire body, not just for the infected area. Only such a complete approach to healing would work, Paracelsus explained. When Froben appeared uncertain, Paracelsus asked, "How badly do you want the leg?" "As much as breath itself," replied Froben, and agreed to follow the healer's instructions to the letter.

Paracelsus first moved the patient from the soft bed where he lay to a straw mattress on the floor. He then ordered Froben's excellent cook to eliminate all rich foods and wines from his employer's menu; the patient would have only simple meals and plenty of juices, herbal teas, and broths. Paracelsus sparingly applied some medication to the infected area. To encourage the reentry of what he called the archaeus, or life force, into the leg, the physician prescribed massage and gentle muscle-tightening exercises. He also insisted that Froben be carried outside to spend part of each day in fresh air and sunshine.

Paracelsus devoted much time to his patient's mental attitude. Whenever Froben began to doubt the success of the treatment, Paracelsus would pour a mysterious powder from the hollow pommel of his sword, mix this "medicine" into a glass of water, and give it to Froben to drink. Although the potion had no taste or odor, it had an immediate tonic effect on Froben. Paracelsus also hired a local entertainer to sing and play the lute for his patient, thus keeping Froben's mind off his illness.

For five days, no improvement was seen. The people of Basel, who were following Froben's fate, began to mur-

The Homeopathic Alternative

For nearly 200 years, patients seeking an alternative to conventional medical treatment have found relief in homeopathy. Homeopaths hold that tiny doses of a substance that causes disease symptoms in a healthy person can cure the symptoms in a sick one.

Homeopathy was founded in the early 1800s by a German physician named Samuel Hahnemann, whose cures inspired a devoted following. His techniques were brought to the U.S. in the 1820s by Swiss and German immigrants, among them a young physician named Constantine Hering. A former skeptic, Hering was won over when a homeopathic remedy saved his infected hand from amputation. He founded three schools of homeopathic medicine;

by the end of the century there were twenty-two of them in the U.S. and more than 100 homeopathic hospitals.

Despite its ongoing popularity (enthusiasts include Queen Elizabeth II, violinist Yehudi Menuhin, and Mother Teresa), homeopathy is scorned by conventional physicians. They ridicule a key tenet, the law of potentization, which states—despite known physical law—that a curative agent's potency increases as it is diluted. Thus homeopaths treat patients with infinitesimally small doses and freely prescribe such toxic substances as snake venom and arsenic; the poisons are so diluted that virtually no trace can be found.

In 1986, French researchers led by Dr. Jacques Benveniste set out to test

Constantine Hering, the Father of American Homeopathy, spent fifty years assembling a massive materia medica of homeopathic remedies.

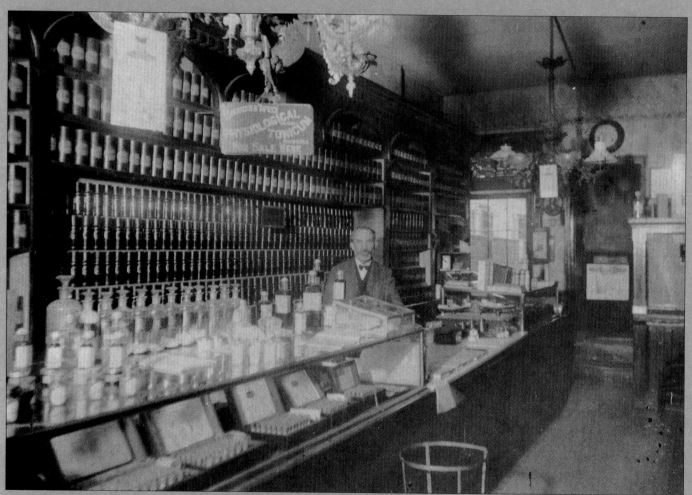

Philadelphian Carl Vischer stands in his pharmacy in 1890, surrounded by bottles containing hundreds of homeopathic nostrums.

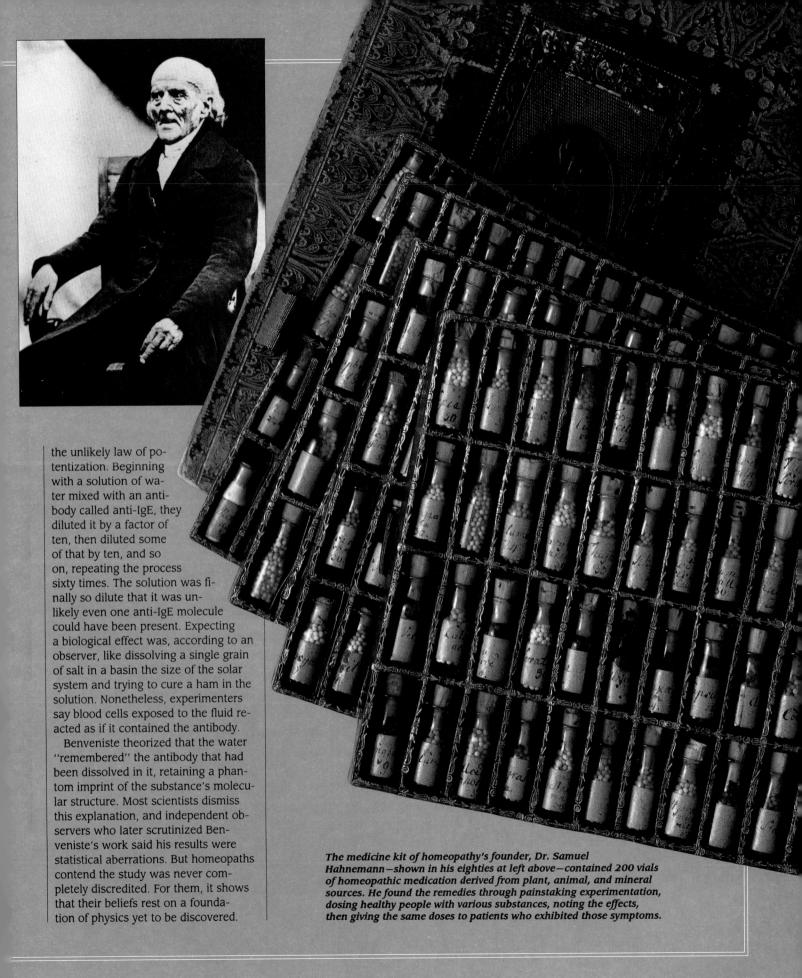

the unlikely law of potentization. Beginning with a solution of water mixed with an antibody called anti-IgE, they diluted it by a factor of ten, then diluted some of that by ten, and so on, repeating the process sixty times. The solution was finally so dilute that it was unlikely even one anti-IgE molecule could have been present. Expecting a biological effect was, according to an observer, like dissolving a single grain of salt in a basin the size of the solar system and trying to cure a ham in the solution. Nonetheless, experimenters say blood cells exposed to the fluid reacted as if it contained the antibody.

Benveniste theorized that the water "remembered" the antibody that had been dissolved in it, retaining a phantom imprint of the substance's molecular structure. Most scientists dismiss this explanation, and independent observers who later scrutinized Benveniste's work said his results were statistical aberrations. But homeopaths contend the study was never completely discredited. For them, it shows that their beliefs rest on a foundation of physics yet to be discovered.

The medicine kit of homeopathy's founder, Dr. Samuel Hahnemann—shown in his eighties at left above—contained 200 vials of homeopathic medication derived from plant, animal, and mineral sources. He found the remedies through painstaking experimentation, dosing healthy people with various substances, noting the effects, then giving the same doses to patients who exhibited those symptoms.

mur that he was in the hands of a charlatan and would surely die. But on the sixth day, Froben's leg was markedly better; for the first time in weeks, he could place the sole of his foot on the floor without pain. By the thirteenth day, he was walking in his garden with a cane. Not only was his leg clearly on the mend, he told his amazed friends, but he had never felt healthier in his life.

At the urging of Froben and Erasmus, Paracelsus was soon named city physician for Basel and professor of medicine at the city's university. But he held these posts only

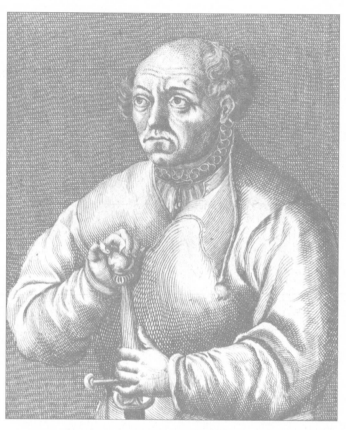

Sixteenth-century Swiss holistic practitioner Paracelsus felt himself superior to such fabled ancient healers as the Roman physician Celsus—hence his name, which means "beyond Celsus."

briefly. His new ideas—and the outspoken, even abrasive manner in which he expressed them—drew the wrath of many in the local medical community, and he was forced to leave the city. From then on, Paracelsus roamed from town to town, giving his medical help to whoever requested it, whether prince or pauper—and in addition to hundreds of paupers, there were no fewer than eighteen princes. His controversial treatments brought him fame and, perhaps, an early death at the age of forty-eight. He died under mysterious circumstances in 1541, some believe at the hands of assassins hired by his physician enemies.

Many medical historians attribute Paracelsus's success to his ability to convince patients that he could cure them. The magical powder from the pommel of his sword, they suggest, was perhaps a sixteenth-century version of the so-called sugar pill—a pharmacologically innocuous substance that has no active effect on the disorder for which it is prescribed. His patients' expectations about the mysterious

medicine, not the powder itself, worked the cure.

Such substances are known as placebos, from the Latin "I shall please." Once overlooked by medical researchers, the placebo effect, as the healing ability of these harmless treatments is called, has become the focus of a number of studies in recent years. Scientists now report that up to forty percent of people suffering from a wide assortment of ailments—from nausea to the common cold—exhibit a lessening of symptoms or a complete cure after taking a placebo. In a major study of patients with angina pectoris—chest pains caused by heart problems—Harvard Medical School cardiologist Herbert Benson compiled results of thirteen surveys made over four decades: Of 1,187 patients who had received placebos, 82 percent demonstrated subjective improvement, and there were objective, medically measurable changes as well.

Just how placebos work their magic remains a mystery, but they appear to generate an emotional reaction that causes physiological changes. When an inert but brightly colored dye is painted on a wart and presented to a patient as a cure, for example, the chemical composition of the skin's surface may actually change, becoming inhospitable to the virus that caused the wart. Placebos can also help repair severely damaged body tissues, such as peptic ulcers, painful open sores on the lining of the stomach or upper part of the small intestine. In a study reported by Dr. Jerome Frank, a psychiatrist at Johns Hopkins University, patients with bleeding peptic ulcers were given injections of distilled water by a doctor who enthusiastically described it as a new

"Every Day in Every Way . . ."

The first modern popularizer of mind-over-body medical techniques was Frenchman Émile Coué, who devised a method of self-healing called autosuggestion.

Born in 1857, Coué discovered the mind's curative powers while studying to be an apothecary. He prescribed a patent medicine to a patient suffering from "an extremely refractory illness." To Coué's amazement, the man immediately recovered. Seeking the source of this miraculous cure, Coué checked the medicine. He found it was a harmless compound, a placebo. He saw at once that the patient's faith in the medicine and in Coué had worked the cure.

Coué went on to study with A. A. Liebeault, who used hypnosis to cure a variety of ailments. Coué concluded that the true power of healing rested with the patient, not the hypnotist. He sought a way for patients to trigger that inner healing ability on their own. Finally, he settled on autosuggestion.

Coué's system was simplicity itself. He told patients to say one phrase several times a day that would put them in a positive, and thus healthful, state of mind. He gave them several phrases to choose from, the most popular being, "Every day in every way I am getting better and better." He believed the best times for invoking the words were the morning and evening, when the unconscious was especially receptive to suggestion.

Autosuggestion soon became a worldwide fad. Coué's patients claimed that his phrases had cured them of everything from asthma to appendicitis. By 1926, the year of Coué's death, hundreds of thousands of people were rising in the morning and going to sleep at night with the hopeful phrases on their lips.

medicine certain to cure them; 70 percent of the patients showed excellent results, lasting more than one year. In contrast, a control group was given the same injection by a nurse who said only that it was an experimental treatment of undetermined effectiveness; scarcely 25 percent of these patients showed improvement.

As this last study suggests, placebos seem to stand as a veritable symbol of the physician's power. Researchers speculate that the placebo administered with the doctor's blessing reduced anxiety and thus lessened the stomach-acid secretions that caused the ulcers. The placebo effect is not always beneficial, however. Patients who fear drugs and distrust doctors often experience nausea, skin eruptions, or other adverse physical reactions after taking a placebo—just as if they had reacted badly to a real medication.

One of the most dramatic and often-cited illustrations of the placebo's power involved a patient with malignant lymphoma, or cancer of the lymphatic glands. As the noted surgeon Dr. Bernard S. Siegel, of Yale New Haven Hospital, describes the case in his 1986 book, *Love, Medicine & Miracles*, the patient, identified only as Mr. Wright, was hospitalized with tumors the size of oranges in his neck, armpits, groin, chest, and abdomen. He was able to breathe only with the aid of an oxygen mask, his spleen and liver were greatly enlarged, and because of a swollen thoracic lymph duct, one to two quarts of milky fluid had to be drained from his chest each day. He was a man on the verge of death.

Lying in his hospital bed waiting to die, Mr. Wright learned about a promising new anticancer drug called Krebiozen, scheduled for clinical tests in the hospital. He pleaded with his doctor to give him the drug. The medication was slated for patients with a life expectancy of three to six months—much longer than Mr. Wright's—but after much deliberation, his wish was granted.

The drug was administered on a Friday. On the following Monday, the doctor returned to the hospital, expecting to find that Mr. Wright's condition had worsened over the weekend. Instead, he encountered a stunning sight: His terminal patient was now walking about the ward, laughing and joking with the nurses. A careful physical examination revealed an even more startling fact—the man's tumors had shrunk by half.

Two weeks later, after additional injections, his body was entirely free of all signs of the disease that had ravaged it for months. Mr. Wright was sent home, seemingly cured.

For two months, he remained in almost perfect health. Then, reports casting doubt on Krebiozen's effectiveness began to appear in the newspapers and on radio and television. Mr. Wright experienced a relapse; his tumors returned.

Suspecting that the placebo effect may have caused both the recovery and the relapse, the doctor set out to convince the patient that the medicine really was effective. He told Mr. Wright to disregard what he had heard. Early shipments of Krebiozen were defective because of storage problems, he explained, but a double-strength version of the drug was to arrive the next day. This new version, the doctor stressed, looked very promising. Hope restored, Mr. Wright eagerly awaited the new drug. To heighten his patient's belief in the medication, the doctor administered the first injection with great fanfare. Unbeknown to the patient, however, the preparation consisted only of distilled water.

Recovery was even more dramatic than before. The tumors disappeared again, and within days the patient was able to return home, where he remained symptom-free for more than two months. Then, the American Medical Association issued its final verdict on Krebiozen, stating that the drug was worthless in the treatment of cancer.

His faith now irrevocably crushed, the patient fell ill again and was readmitted to the hospital. He died less than two days later.

The placebo effect depends on a patient's conscious

Healing by the Divine Mind

To frail, sickly Mary Baker Glover Patterson, the circular that arrived at her Concord, New Hampshire, home in 1861 brought a ray of hope into a singularly unfortunate life. Impoverished, trapped in an unhappy second marriage (after having been widowed at the age of twenty-three), and afflicted since childhood with a host of ailments ranging from chronic headaches, fatigue, and depression to severe spinal pain, the forty-year-old woman read the pamphlet eagerly.

It described the healing work of mesmerist Phineas P. Quimby *(page 91)* and the cures he achieved without medicines. Having lost faith in traditional physicians, who had failed to alleviate her suffering, Mrs. Patterson was determined to meet Quimby. Pinching her pennies, she saved enough by October 1862 to travel to Quimby's Portland, Maine, offices—a journey that would lead not only to her own cure but to the founding of a new religion: Christian Science.

Years later, Mary Baker Eddy—as she was known after a divorce and new marriage—wrote that she felt better as soon as she entered his office. He laid his hands on her head and said her illness was all in her mind. A week later, she was so robust she climbed the 182 steps to the dome of Portland's city hall.

Quimby believed he had discovered the secret of Jesus Christ's healing ministry—that the mind was the key to healing. He called it the Science of Health, or the Science of Christ, and his new patient became a tireless promulgator of this view. She advertised her services as a healer in the Quimby mold. At the same time, she worked feverishly on what was to become her central philosophical and theological treatise, *Science and Health,* a tome that borrowed heavily from Quimby's own writings and terminology.

But by 1875, when *Science and Health* was published, Mrs. Eddy downplayed Quimby's influence, insisting that her beliefs were divine revelations. In fact, Mrs. Eddy differed sharply from her old mentor in that she believed it was not the human mind that cured disease, but the mind of God. To her, the divine mind was the governing principle of the universe, as unvarying, as "scientific," as mathematical law. Disease was a product of the mortal mind, in effect a scientific error that could be eradicated only by coming to know God's mind through prayer.

These theories were firmly rooted in the New England Calvinist tradition equating sin and sickness, as well as the more ancient Christian belief in the healing power of prayer. But Mrs. Eddy was considered highly radical by conventional churches because of what appeared to be a *reducto ad absurdum* in her thinking: her view that illness and disease, along with all physical matter, were merely illusions that did not exist except in the human mind.

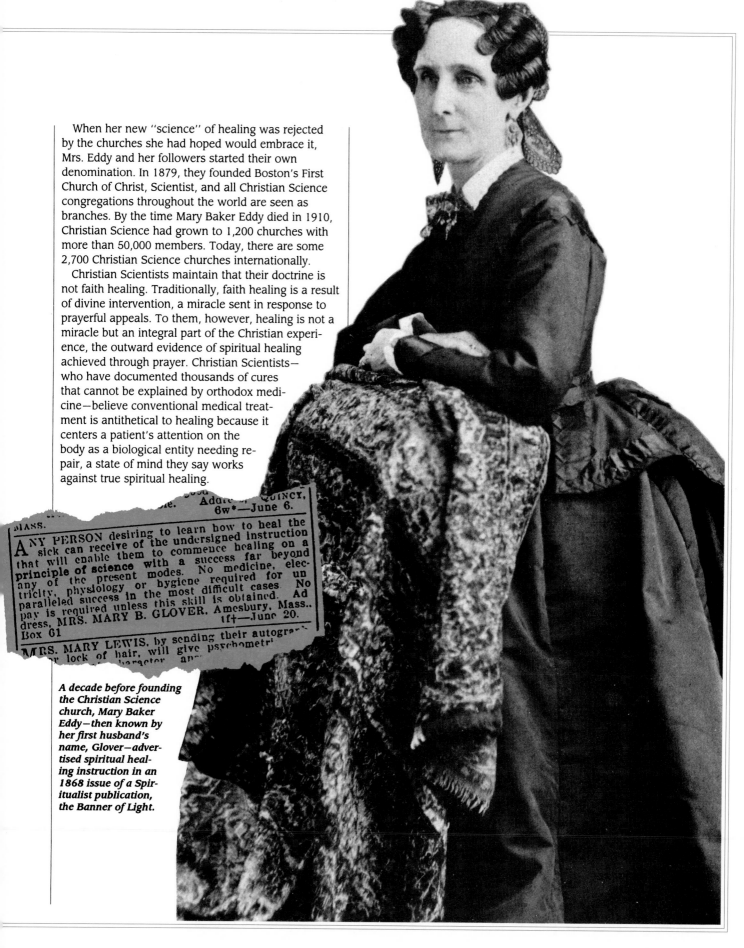

When her new "science" of healing was rejected by the churches she had hoped would embrace it, Mrs. Eddy and her followers started their own denomination. In 1879, they founded Boston's First Church of Christ, Scientist, and all Christian Science congregations throughout the world are seen as branches. By the time Mary Baker Eddy died in 1910, Christian Science had grown to 1,200 churches with more than 50,000 members. Today, there are some 2,700 Christian Science churches internationally.

Christian Scientists maintain that their doctrine is not faith healing. Traditionally, faith healing is a result of divine intervention, a miracle sent in response to prayerful appeals. To them, however, healing is not a miracle but an integral part of the Christian experience, the outward evidence of spiritual healing achieved through prayer. Christian Scientists—who have documented thousands of cures that cannot be explained by orthodox medicine—believe conventional medical treatment is antithetical to healing because it centers a patient's attention on the body as a biological entity needing repair, a state of mind they say works against true spiritual healing.

> QUINCY,
> MASS. Addre.
> 6w*—June 6.
>
> ANY PERSON desiring to learn how to heal the sick can receive of the undersigned instruction that will enable them to commence healing on a principle of science with a success far beyond any of the present modes. No medicine, electricity, physiology or hygiene required for unparalleled success in the most difficult cases. No pay is required unless this skill is obtained. Address, MRS. MARY B. GLOVER, Amesbury, Mass.. Box 61 tf†—June 20.
>
> MRS. MARY LEWIS, by sending their autogra~ r lock of hair, will give psychometr' ~aracter an~

A decade before founding the Christian Science church, Mary Baker Eddy—then known by her first husband's name, Glover—advertised spiritual healing instruction in an 1868 issue of a Spiritualist publication, the Banner of Light.

belief that he or she is undergoing some kind of beneficial treatment. Yet the unconscious mind—the part to which people have no direct access—may also influence a person's state of health, as research into psychosomatic illnesses is showing.

A psychosomatic illness is one that is induced or influenced by the mind, usually as the result of some kind of emotional stress. This is not to say that the illness is "all in the head," for the symptoms of a psychosomatic ailment can be very real, from high blood pressure to skin rashes and painful headaches. Unlike other illnesses, however, one that is psychosomatic has no direct organic cause, such as a virus or a physical injury.

Scientists believe psychosomatic illnesses are connected with the primitive fight-or-flight reaction, an arousal response that occurs in all animals when confronted with danger. The reaction provides the body with extra energy and prepares it to either combat a situation or flee from it. Characteristics of the fight-or-flight reaction include a tensing of the muscles, a rise in blood pressure and heart rate, a sharpening of the senses, and a boost in the production of adrenaline, a stimulative hormone.

For primitive humans, the major events, or stressors, that set off the fight-or-flight reaction were physical threats that could quickly be resolved by decisive action—fleeing from a fierce animal, for example, or hurrying to shelter in the face of a storm. Danger behind it, the body soon resumed its normal functioning.

Today, however, stressors are more likely to be emotional than physical and are not so readily dealt with. A stressor can be an everyday event that triggers anger or frustration, such as losing the car keys or encountering a traffic jam on the way to work. Or it can be a major crisis, such as divorce or the death of a loved one. But the stressor itself is not as important to health as the reaction to it. If a person learns to cope with the stressor in a positive manner—accepting the inevitability of arriving late, for instance, or mourning the deceased—the body regains its equilibri-

um. If the problem nags on unconfronted, however, the arousal reaction can persist, causing anxiety, tension, helplessness, and depression. It is this latter response that leads to stress-related disorders.

Psychosomatic illnesses are quite common. General practitioners report that one-half to three-quarters of the patients visiting their offices complain of symptoms that are clearly stress related. Usually, the person suffering from a psychosomatic illness is unaware of its connection to a repressed emotion. A man whose job is threatened, for example, probably does not realize that the painful ache in his lower back may be a direct physiological response to his fear of being fired.

A common psychosomatic illness is irritable bowel syndrome, a condition that afflicts millions of people but for which no organic cause has been found. Although the symptoms—which include abdominal pain and either diarrhea or constipation—are real enough, no physical damage to the colon occurs and the condition is never life threatening. Stressful emotions appear to be a major cause. Attacks often take place after a stress-evoking event, such as an argument with a friend or a financial setback. Worrying about an attack also can bring one on.

Yet another common psychosomatic complaint is the tension headache—a dull, steady ache or feeling of tightness on both sides of the head that can last for hours, weeks, even months. Usually, no other physical symptom accompanies the headache, aside from a stiff neck or a clenched jaw. Stress is believed to be the source of most tension headaches. It sets off the fight-or-flight reaction in the brain, which in turn causes muscles throughout the body to contract. If the tension continues unabated, muscles in the neck, head, and face begin to send messages of pain through the nerves to the brain, and a full-blown tension headache begins.

One aspect of psychosomatic illness that has stirred interest in medical circles is the notion that certain personality types are predisposed to specific ailments. Systematic studies have sought a link between personality and illness.

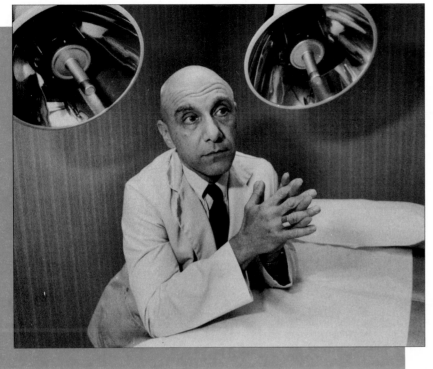

Rx for Love and Miracles

In the early 1970s, Dr. Bernard S. Siegel, a successful Connecticut surgeon and cancer specialist, had come to view his patients "as machines I had to repair." Disenchanted, he considered becoming a veterinarian, "because veterinarians can hug their patients." But instead he humanized his practice, embracing the people he treated, urging them to call him "Bernie," and crying and laughing with them. He also began to explore the roles that hope, love, and spirituality play in healing.

In 1978, Siegel founded a therapy group called ECaP, for Exceptional Cancer Patients. Its members were encouraged to participate aggressively in their own therapy by asking questions, expressing their emotions, and marshaling positive feelings. Siegel was amazed at the results. As he related in his 1986 bestseller, *Love, Medicine & Miracles*, "People whose conditions had been stable or deteriorating for a long time suddenly began to get well before my eyes." Such seemingly inexplicable spontaneous remissions are usually seen as medical anomalies. But to Siegel they show a fundamental link between bodily health and the mind. Critics say his approach places an unfair burden on patients, but he insists that where illness is concerned, "attitude is all-important."

Some researchers regard the approach as fruitless. As early as 1953, Dr. Lawrence S. Kubie, of the New York Psychoanalytic Institute, examined patients suffering from migraines, ulcerative colitis, and heart disease but uncovered no consistent personality types. "I have been impressed by the dissimilarities at least as vividly as by the similarities," he concluded.

Yet some evidence seems to link personality with disease. People who suffer from irritable bowel syndrome, for example, have been found to be tense, anxious, emotionally unpredictable, busy, and often hurried. Interestingly, victims of this illness can be divided even further along personality lines: Those who suffer mostly from constipation tend to respond to emotional arousal with anger, tension, and defensiveness, while those who have problems with diarrhea are more likely to react to similar situations with feelings of hopelessness and despair.

Research suggests that personality may play a role in other illnesses as well. One of the most complete studies to address this theory was conducted in 1957 by psychiatrist Floyd O. Ring at the University of Nebraska College of Medicine. Ring set up personality interviews with more than 400 patients referred to him by medical colleagues. To participate in the study, a patient had to suffer from one of fourteen ailments, including high blood pressure, peptic ulcers, rheumatoid arthritis, asthma, diabetes, and blocked coronary arteries.

Each interview lasted between fifteen and twenty-five minutes. To ensure that Ring and the other examiners received no clues about the illnesses of the study subjects, the patients were instructed to avoid discussing any symptom, treatment, disability, or other potentially revealing aspect of their physical condition. In addition, each patient's body was covered during the interview so the examiners would not receive any visual clues. If either of these safeguards failed—even if a hand slipped out from under the cover—the patient was excluded from the final findings of the study.

A Rebirth of Positive Feelings

The expressions playing across the face of the woman on the left in these photographs show her intense emotions as she undergoes a process called Vivation. For two hours, the woman (called a viver) lies wrapped in a blanket while the "Vivation professional" at her side coaches her in a breathing technique that helps her relax and release deeply suppressed feelings.

Practitioners say we all harbor hidden negative feelings, the residue of unpleasant experiences. During Vivation, these feelings are relived in a pleasurable context, which transforms them into positive emotions. The viver does not always recall the original circumstances but reexperiences the sensation and, in the process, comes to feel ecstatic and alive (or vivacious).

Created by Californian Jim Leonard, who trademarked the name in 1987, Vivation grew out of a therapeutic process called rebirthing, developed in the early 1970s. Rebirthing participants try to re-create their own births in order to reexperience the emotions. In reliving that primal trauma, they get it out of their system, in effect. Neither Vivation nor rebirthing is designed specifically to heal illness, but believers feel that suppressed negative emotions have an adverse effect on the body and mind and that their release enhances well-being.

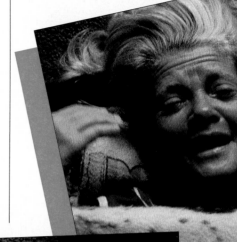

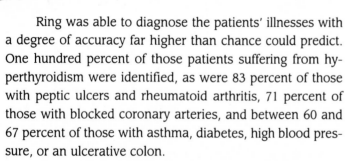

Ring was able to diagnose the patients' illnesses with a degree of accuracy far higher than chance could predict. One hundred percent of those patients suffering from hyperthyroidism were identified, as were 83 percent of those with peptic ulcers and rheumatoid arthritis, 71 percent of those with blocked coronary arteries, and between 60 and 67 percent of those with asthma, diabetes, high blood pressure, or an ulcerative colon.

One of the questions Ring asked participants was, "If you were sitting on a park bench and a stranger just your size, age, and sex walked up and kicked you in the shins, what would you do?" Answers divided the subjects into three main categories. Those who responded that they would immediately strike back were categorized by Ring as "excessive reactors." Although overly apprehensive, they had little difficulty expressing their thoughts and tended to react freely to feelings of fear or anger. People in this group of patients, Ring noted, were most likely to have degenerative arthritis, peptic ulcers, or coronary occlusion.

Those who said they would do nothing if kicked in the shins by a stranger were placed in the category of "deficient reactors." According to Ring, these patients tended to suppress their true emotions and, therefore, to refrain from acting on them. He found this group most likely to suffer from

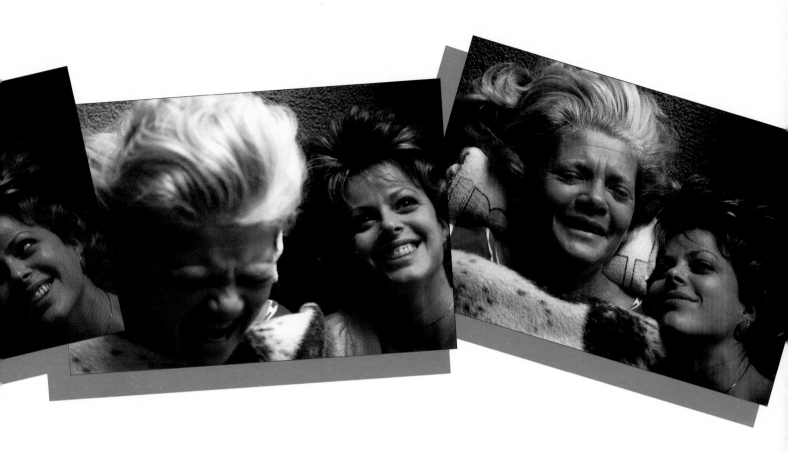

skin rashes, rheumatoid arthritis, or ulcerative colitis.

The final group were "restrained reactors." Although aware of their feelings of fear and anger, they seldom expressed them openly. Their typical response to the question about being kicked in the shin was, "I'd be pretty mad" or "I might hit him." Most of the patients in this group suffered from asthma, diabetes, high blood pressure, hyperthyroidism, or migraine headaches.

To be sure, psychosomatic problems are not restricted to actual illness. At New York's Columbia Presbyterian Medical Center, in the early 1940s, Dr. Helen Flanders Dunbar conducted studies of people who suffered numerous mishaps—the accident-prone—and found a distinct personality type: They appeared generally healthy, intelligent, and cheerful but had an unstable, cavalier attitude about work and personal relationships. Their marriages were often casual, and they tended to be resentful of authority and given to impulsive outbursts of undirected energy.

Another, less common, psychosomatic condition, termed autoerythrocyte sensitization, involves a spontaneous bruising of the skin. Women are the usual victims; they feel sudden pain in a part of the body, followed by swelling and severe discoloration. The bruises can be extremely large, and the sufferers often experience headaches, fainting spells, and numbness. In an early study of the phenom-

enon, Harvard physicians Frank Gardner and Louis Diamond found that most people with spontaneous bruising had at one time experienced a grave trauma, such as being hit by a car, and apparently developed an autoimmune reaction to their own red blood cells.

According to David P. Agle, a psychiatrist at Case Western Reserve University Medical School in Cleveland, "Episodes of spontaneous bruising are frequently related to emotionally stressful situations." One woman happened to see a bullet wound above the right knee of a man who resembled her brother; she soon developed a painful bruise in the same area. Another woman experienced a major bruise on the back of her right hand after she repressed a powerful urge to strike an annoying person. She later suffered a second episode, involving her leg, that was so incapacitating she was hospitalized for several weeks.

In rare cases, although the skin is not broken, blood actually oozes from the victim's hair follicles. Researchers speculate that this phenomenon may account for those people down through the centuries who have appeared to suffer the wounds of Christ—the religious stigmatics, mostly women, who spontaneously bleed from their hands, feet, shoulders, sides, and scalp.

To explore further the mind-body connection and its

effect on health, medical researchers and social scientists have joined forces in recent years in a new field of study called psychoneuroimmunology, or PNI. Research in PNI focuses on the subtle connections between the brain and the immune system—a term for all the parts and functions of the body that fight off invading organisms.

Until the mid-1970s, scientists were under the impression that the immune system worked independently of the brain and, certainly, of the emotions. Then, in 1974, there came a pioneering study by University of Rochester psychologist Robert Ader. Originally, the study was to be a relatively simple taste-aversion experiment. Ader gave laboratory rats a saccharine solution to drink, then immediately injected them with cyclophosphamide, a drug that is known to cause severe stomach pains. After only one injection, most of the rats learned to associate the sweet taste of the saccharine water with the discomforting cramps and to avoid the saccharine. When the conditioned rats were forced to take additional doses of saccharine without injec-

tions of cyclophosphamide, they continued to sicken and some even died.

Upon closer examination of the drug, Ader learned that cyclophosphamide, in addition to inducing stomach distress, was capable of suppressing the immune system, which could have produced the rats' illnesses. But could a few doses—or even a single dose—of the drug leave the animals so vulnerable to disease? He doubted it.

Ader wondered if something else might be happening: Perhaps the rats had become conditioned not only to experience pain after drinking the saccharine, but to suppress their immune system as well. Working with immunologist Nicholas Cohen of the University of Rochester, Ader set out to test this hypothesis by repeating the experiment with three new groups of rats, using two groups as controls. He discovered that his guess was right—once conditioned as before, rats fed saccharine continued to lower their immunological defenses and thus weakened their resistance to disease, even when not given immunosuppressors. In other

Psychologist Robert Ader explains how in 1974 he discovered a way to condition rats to suppress their immune systems. His experiments demonstrated a link between the immune system and the psyche, long viewed as separate from one another.

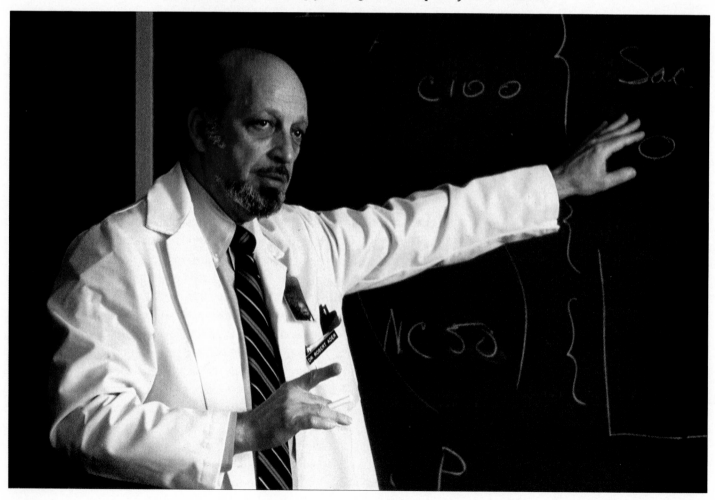

words, it appeared that, at least in laboratory rats, the mind could influence the body's susceptibility to disease.

Ader's study spawned the now-exploding field of PNI research and with it a greater understanding of the immune system. Unlike the cardiovascular system with its clearly connected heart and blood vessels or the nervous system with its brain, spinal cord, and nerves, the immune system's work is primarily done by an assortment of cells and molecules scattered throughout the body. Most common are certain white blood cells, or lymphocytes, that prowl the bloodstream, looking for foreign intruders known as antigens. When they discover an intruder—say, a bacterium—they attach themselves to it and release antibodies designed to

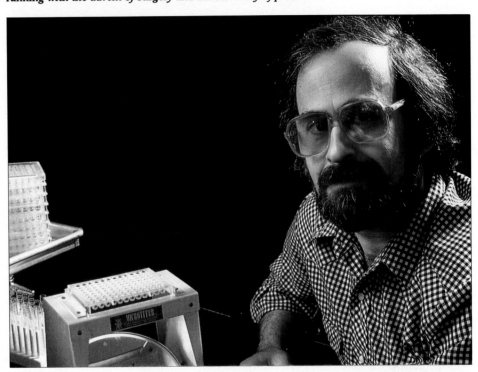

Immunologist Nicholas Cohen, pictured here with samples of rats' blood, collaborated with Robert Ader (opposite) on the breakthrough studies that opened the field of psychoneuroimmunology, the study of the connection between the mind and the immune system. PNI, as it is less cumbersomely known, has since been characterized by a number of scientists as a "third revolution" in Western medicine, ranking with the advent of surgery and the discovery of penicillin.

destroy the invader from within. Other major blood cell types that make up the immune system's arsenal include macrophages, large scavenger cells that arrive after lymphocytes to "eat up" weakened antigens, and natural killer cells, which are known as NKs, whose specialty is fighting viruses and tumors.

Sometimes, the immune system overreacts to an antigen, producing the all-too-common allergic reaction. Hay fever, for example, results when the immune system sends too many of its troops out to respond to the harmless ragweed pollen. At other times, the immune system may break down and begin to attack healthy cells. The result is an autoimmune disease, such as rheumatoid arthritis, pernicious anemia, or systemic lupus erythematosus (SLE), a disorder that usually attacks young women and is capable, in its extreme forms, of producing mental changes, kidney damage, and even death.

More commonly, however, the immune system simply becomes suppressed—as it did with Ader's rats—opening

the way for viruses, bacteria, and other toxins to invade and take over the body. If the immune system remains suppressed and does not fight back, death can result. People with AIDS, or acquired immune deficiency syndrome, have immune systems so weak that their bodies eventually become targets for opportunistic infections and cancer.

Just what causes the immune system to go askew is not completely understood, but the brain is most certainly involved. A study undertaken in the late 1970s by neuroscientist Karen Bulloch, now at the University of California, San Diego, revealed direct neurological pathways between the brain and the immune system. Later studies confirmed that the two apparently "talk" to each other. The brain sends chemical messages to the immune system that appear to influence the activity of the lymphocytes. The immune system, in turn, feeds its own chemical messages back to an area of the brain known as the hypothalamus, which is very much involved with emotions, responding to them and regulating their physical effects.

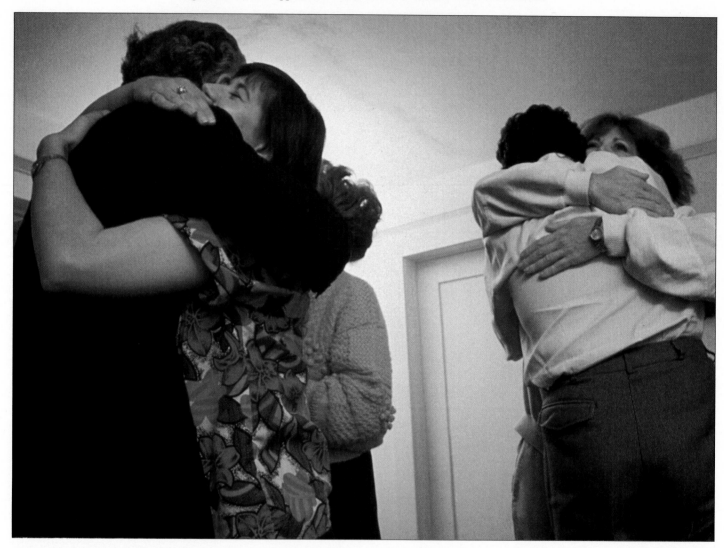

Cancer patients embrace one another at the Wellness Community in Santa Monica, California, an organization inspired in part by the residential programs used to treat drug abusers. The community was founded in 1982 by retired attorney Harold H. Benjamin, whose wife's battle against breast cancer taught him that isolation could be physically harmful to a patient and that "camaraderie, togetherness, and support" could enhance conventional medical treatment.

Given this two-way feedback system, it seems reasonable—as PNI researchers now believe—that the same emotions that affect the hypothalamus may also affect the immune system. Research has shown that chronic stress causes the brain to release into the body a host of hormones that are potent inhibitors of the immune system. These chemicals suppress the system by reducing the number of lymphocytes, macrophages, and NK cells circulating in the body.

This may explain why people experience increased rates of infection, cancer, arthritis, and many other ailments after losing a spouse. In a 1975 study of the effects of bereavement, Dr. R. W. Bartrop and his associates in Australia compared blood samples from grieving spouses with control samples taken from people who were not bereaved. Often the blood samples of the bereaved showed a much lower level of lymphocyte activity than was present in the control group's samples. Emotional factors also seem to slow production of tumor-fighting NK cells in women with breast cancer. In one breast-cancer study, begun in 1981 by

132

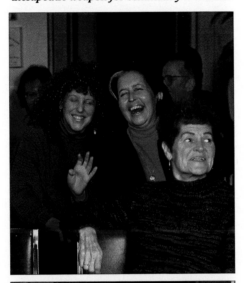

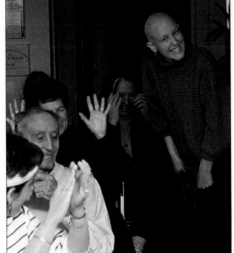

Sandra Levy, a psychologist at the Pittsburgh Cancer Institute, low-NK activity was found to be "significantly associated" with the spread of the cancer. Levy came to the conclusion that more than half of the fluctuating NK levels were the result of psychological factors, such as how the patient coped with stress and whether or not she felt she had the support of friends and family in her fight against the disease.

Being under almost any kind of stress can weaken the immune system. But an individual's attitude toward stress may determine whether the system breaks down. People who chronically feel that their lives are out of control appear to have more difficulty fighting off illness than those who are hopeful and positive about life.

In one study, published in 1971 by researchers at the University of Rochester Medical Center, sixty-eight women who had undergone biopsies for cervical cancer—but did not yet know the results—were interviewed to determine their attitudes of hopefulness or helplessness. Of the women, twenty-eight turned out to have cancer and forty did not. Based solely on the interviews, researchers correctly predicted cancer in nineteen of the women who actually had the disease (an accuracy rate of 68 percent) and predicted negative results for thirty-one of the forty who indeed were found to be cancer-free (an accuracy rate of 77 percent). The women who spoke most positively about their lives, the results showed, were least likely to have the cancer.

Helplessness can become a learned response, according to University of Pennsylvania research psychologist Martin Seligman, who began studying this phenomenon in 1967. Laboratory rats subjected to electric shocks and given no means of escape became so apathetic that they failed to take advantage of an exit even when one was provided. People, too, can become so conditioned to pessimistic feelings that they miss opportunities to improve their lives. In another of Seligman's experiments, human test subjects were deprived of the ability to control the noise level in a laboratory where they were confined. Later, when an irritatingly bright light was added to the room, about two-thirds of the subjects failed to adjust its intensity, although they had the power to do so. They had become conditioned to believe that they were helpless.

Being without a strong support network of friends and relatives may also be detrimental to the immune system. In one of the largest studies of the effect of loneliness on death rates, researchers found that people with the fewest close relationships were three times more likely to die prematurely than others of the same age and sex. In fact, some scientists now cite social isolation as "a major risk factor" for death, perhaps as much of a risk as cigarette smoking. The study cited similar findings among nursing home residents, whose lives are often lonely.

The story of Roseto, Pennsylvania, a small slate-quarrying town of fewer than 2,000 inhabitants, illustrates the important effect that social interactions can have on health. Some years ago, epidemiologists went to Roseto to uncover the secret behind the town's very low rate of death from coronary heart disease. Expecting to find a populace

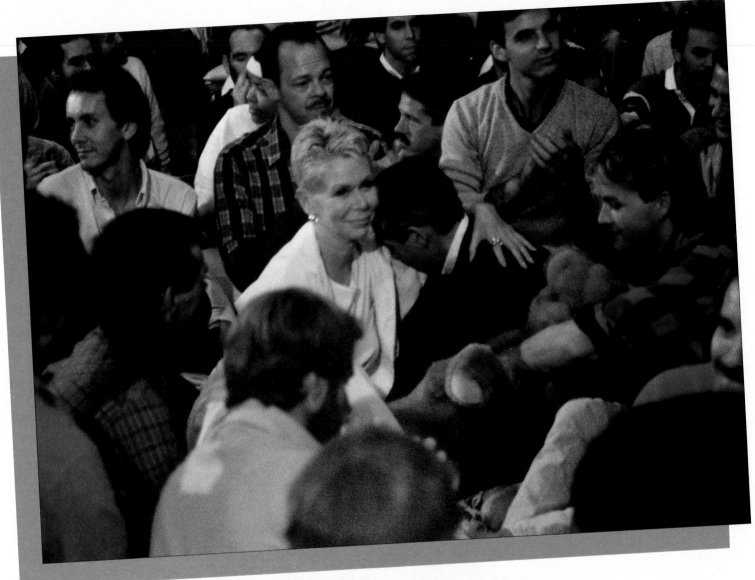

Louise Hay embraces an AIDS patient at a Hayride support group. Believing AIDS to be a disease of self-hatred—an emotion that she contends weakens the immune system— Hay espouses a "loving treatment," giving patients unconditional affection and acceptance.

with exemplary health habits, the researchers were surprised to discover that just the opposite was true. The people of Roseto had the same deplorable habits as the citizens of most other communities. They smoked too much, ate too much, and exercised too little. What, then, accounted for the lower mortality rate? Apparently, protection came from the town's close sense of community. In Roseto, families knew and cared about each other. They shared in each other's triumphs and troubles, joys and sadnesses. Someone was always available to help out when needed or simply to lend a sympathetic ear.

Further research showed that when people moved out of Roseto and left this supportive network of friends behind, their heart attack rates climbed, eventually becoming comparable to national levels. Social support was more impor-

tant in predicting heart disease for the people of Roseto than any other factor.

Recognizing the importance of a caring environment, many doctors are now urging patients with serious illnesses to join with others who are in similar circumstances. These groups relieve the isolation felt by many people and encourage the development of positive attitudes. Since 1982, for example, individuals with cancer have regularly attended meetings in a yellow wooden house in Santa Monica, California, home to a self-help group known as the Wellness Community, which was described by one participant as an "extended family." Group members share the stories of their lives and illnesses, exchange tips about coping with chemotherapy and radiation treatments, and—perhaps most important—help each other laugh and feel hopeful about the future. One of the group's regular and most popular activities is the Joke Fest, when members tell funny stories, including outrageous ones about cancer, to the huge delight of the others.

Taking the group therapy concept one step further, and emerging as one of the leaders in the field, is Louise L. Hay of Santa Monica, California. Hay's own life story includes a childhood of abuse, a traumatic marriage breakup, and a fearsome, but successful, bout with cancer. In addition to advocating group support for those with devastating illnesses, Hay tirelessly promotes a loving attitude and affirmative thought patterns as the path to health and defense against all manner of disease. "The thoughts we think and the words we speak create our life experiences, including our illnesses," she claims. "Release the *need* in your life for your condition and your illness can disappear."

Many are listening to Louise Hay; her book *Heal Your Body,* offering positive thoughts to use against hundreds of afflictions from acne and abdominal cramps to glaucoma, frigidity, fungus, incontinence, and warts, has sold more than 400,000 copies in ten languages. In 1985, Hay started a support group for AIDS patients and their loved ones, offering hope and self-respect and counseling that "love is the most powerful stimulant to the immune system." Within a few years, she was holding weekly sessions, or Hayrides, as she likes to call them, for 600 to 700 AIDS sufferers at a West Hollywood auditorium. Participants described the sessions to a *Los Angeles Times* reporter in 1988 as "the most joyful place in town on any Wednesday night."

To the medical community, Hay is a controversial figure. Many physicians agree that her brand of counseling can be uplifting to those patients who previously found little in their predicaments to give them hope. But many medical experts find the claim that a lack of love in one's life or low self-esteem may bring on AIDS, as Hay states in *Heal Your Body,* far-fetched at the very least—some would say ludicrous. "As a physician," said Dr. Michael Gottlieb, the AIDS specialist who first pinpointed the disease as a threatening new medical syndrome, "I think that love and acceptance

and forgiveness may well be an important component of healing, but AIDS is a viral disease caused by a virus and not by a lack of love."

Medical practitioners also point out a dark side to the notion that the individual is solely responsible, through thoughts and words, for his or her own health. As Dr. Peter Wolfe, an assistant clinical professor of medicine at UCLA who also treats people with AIDS, puts it, "The flip side is that if people get sick, they tend to blame themselves for getting sick and I don't think that's very healthy."

Hay admits that her message is not grounded in science and, when pointedly questioned, explains that what she terms "healing" occurs on many levels—psychological as well as physical—and does not necessarily mean "cure." Although a number of AIDS patients attending her sessions have died from their disease, others maintain they have been cured of the deadly virus. Most medical experts would attribute these cases to long-term remission or false positive results on the individual's initial test.

Developing warm and caring friendships is just one way cancer and AIDS patients and others are learning to positively affect their outlooks if not their immune systems. Other techniques involve more solitary pursuits that focus on using the brain to gain control over the body. One such technique is biological feedback, or biofeedback, as it is commonly called. This is a technique, based on relaxation, that helps patients learn to gain control over such involuntary physiological phenomena as heartbeat, blood pressure, brain waves, and body temperature. Biofeedback has been notably successful in helping people overcome a variety of ailments, including migraine headaches, hypertension, irregular heartbeat, and even mild epilepsy.

Biofeedback is accomplished with the help of specially designed machines that gather biological information from patients while simultaneously feeding it back to them in a form they can either see or hear. Muscle tension, for example, can be signaled by a flashing light or the sound of a beeper. The participants first learn to identify the signal and

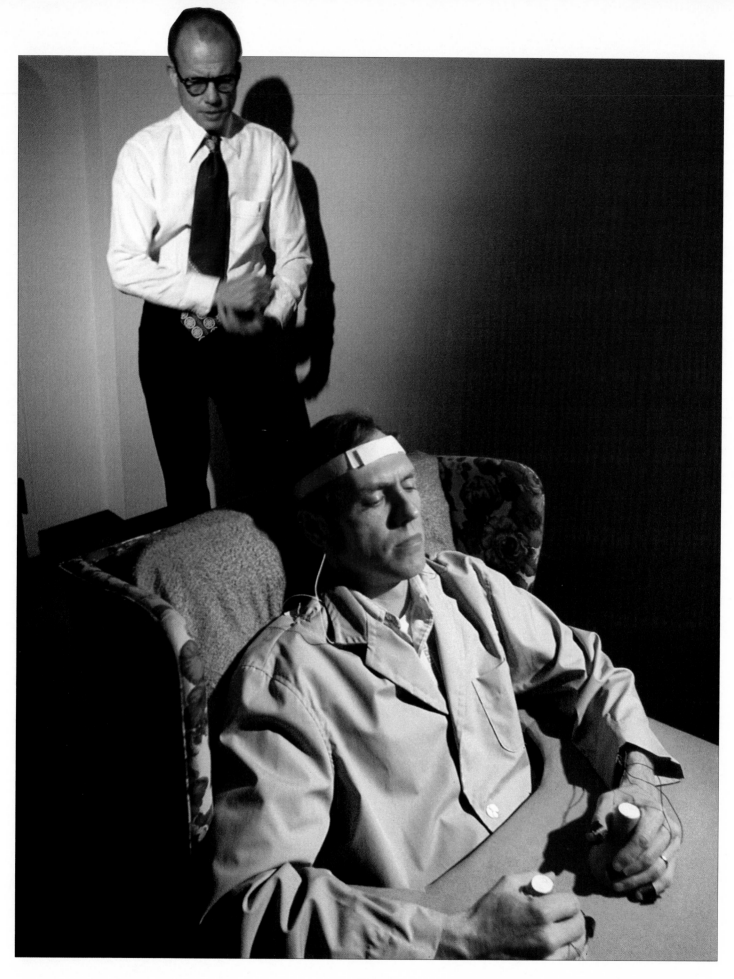

then, through trial and error, how to control the function that triggers it. The constant feedback of information enables them to ascertain immediately whether their attempts at control have been successful. Once they have mastered these skills in a supervised setting, they are taught the more difficult task of using their regulatory techniques in everyday situations.

Biofeedback can provide some surprising information about sources of stress. Most patients are amazed to discover, for example, how variable their heartbeat is. At first, as they watch their heart trace patterns on an electrocardiograph, they tend to believe that the rhythm is random. Then they realize that the heart is actually responding to the slightest movement of their bodies. Breathing deeply or sitting upright, for example, causes the heart rate to decelerate, while rapid, shallow breaths or slouching speeds it up. The patients soon begin to recognize that thoughts can also influence the beat of the heart. When someone remembers a relaxing vacation, the heart rate slows down, but when he or she thinks about a stressful experience—such as a work deadline or an argument with a friend—the heart tends to pump faster.

Finally, as the biofeedback work progresses, the participants gain an even deeper understanding of the relationship between mind and body. They begin to realize that by projecting feelings of warmth and heaviness into the heart area, they can cause their pulses to decelerate. Or, conversely, by projecting cool, tight sensations to the same area, they can cause an acceleration in heartbeat. When this awareness has been reached, participants are ready to use these sensations outside the laboratory to confront and control the way their bodies react to stress.

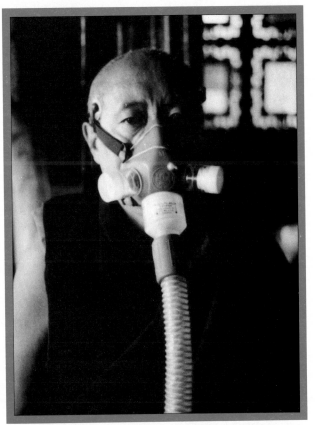

In an experiment by Dr. Herbert Benson, a respirator measures a Buddist monk's oxygen consumption during deep meditation. The results revealed that meditation could reduce the body's metabolic rate.

Experts advise that for biofeedback training to be successful, it must be done in a quiet, serene setting and under the care of a skilled instructor who will provide continuous reinforcement and support. Only in such a stressless environment, they contend, can one truly learn how to respond to stress. Once the process is mastered, however, adepts can relax their bodies totally.

In this respect, biofeedback has much in common with yoga and other traditional Eastern forms of meditation *(pages 70-71)*. In meditation, one's attention is also focused inward, sometimes on a particular word, known as a mantra, sometimes on the rhythm of breathing. Both the body and mind are withdrawn from external stimulation. The key to successful meditation is the same as for biofeedback—a letting go of the anxiety, tension, and negative thoughts that crowd daily life. Eventually, the mind drifts into a mild trancelike state, sometimes called the alpha state, in which brain waves, as measured by an electroencephalograph, slow down to a frequency between eight and twelve cycles per second.

Meditation offers the body many physical benefits. It can lower blood pressure, pulse rate, and the levels of stress hormones in the blood. It can also raise the body's pain threshold. And researchers are exploring possible uses of meditation or relaxation techniques in reducing insulin dependence among diabetics and in raising the quantity of important immune system cells in the blood.

Other techniques for relaxation have also proved beneficial in reversing or reducing the harmful physiological effects of stress. One early method, called progressive relaxation, was developed by University of Chicago psychophysiologist Edmund Jacobson in the 1930s. After noting that most people are unaware that their muscles tense during times of stress, Jacobson designed a method of alternately contracting and relaxing various muscle groups, such as those in the arm or neck, so that a subject becomes more aware of how each state feels. The individual can then learn to recognize stress in its early stages and respond by relaxing the appropriate muscles.

Another method, developed in the 1920s by the German psychiatrist J. H. Schultz, combined Western techniques of self-suggestion with ancient yoga. Called autogenic training, this two-pronged approach is still practiced today. Students undergo weeks of instruction during which they are taught to repeat key phrases, such as "my right arm is heavy" or "my right arm is warm," while in a passive, quiet state, until the sensation of warmth or heaviness—and relaxation—takes over the body.

Once the relaxation segment is mastered, the trainee learns to pair the meditation with another component, known as visualization, or guided imagery. Visualization is an attempt to prompt the body to do consciously what it usually does unconsciously: fight disease. The technique, which seems to be especially effective in promoting physical healing, is thought to accomplish its goal by fooling the body into thinking a vivid mental image is the same as a physical experience.

The young rocketeer who apparently used his imaginary starship to blast away his brain cancer became an expert at visualization. So did a patient hospitalized with a seemingly hopeless bladder cancer, whose case has been reported by Elmer and Alyce Green of the Menninger Clinic's psychophysiology laboratory. The man's doctors hypnotized him, then asked him to find the room in his brain that contained all the valves that controlled the blood supply to his body. Next they instructed the patient to shut off the valve that supplied blood to his cancer. The man indicated that he had found the source and closed it. Indeed, his condition improved so dramatically that he was allowed to leave the hospital, returning only for periodic checkups. During one such examination, however, a mishap with a

Cell biologist Joan Borysenko teaches guided imagery in her Mind/ Body Clinic at Boston's New England Deaconess Hospital, encouraging the patient to create a mental picture of his immune system battling disease. In one study, patients who received such training as part of a disease-fighting strategy that also included nutrition counseling and yoga reduced their physical symptoms by 22 percent.

diagnostic instrument caused the patient's death; an autopsy revealed that his cancer had shrunk from the size of a grapefruit to that of a golf ball.

Other cancer patients learn to "see" the malignant cancer cells in their bodies and then to imagine those cells being engulfed and destroyed by the body's unflagging heroes, the cells of the immune system. Some patients have come up with extremely creative images. Actress and comedian Gilda Radner, for example, developed several visualization fantasies to help in her battle against ovarian cancer. One fantasy had her lymphocytes jumping up and down and singing, "Ding, dong, the witch is dead!" In another, she cast the cancer cells as menacing motorcyclists who litter a beach—Radner's body—with beer cans and cigarette butts, and the lymphocytes as healthy, suntanned surfers who chase the bad guys off the sand.

Some experiments have indicated that imaging may actually raise the level of lymphocytes and other immune system cells in the blood. After one year of imagery sessions, ten cancer patients in a Maryland study showed an increase in white blood cells, which attacked invading or-

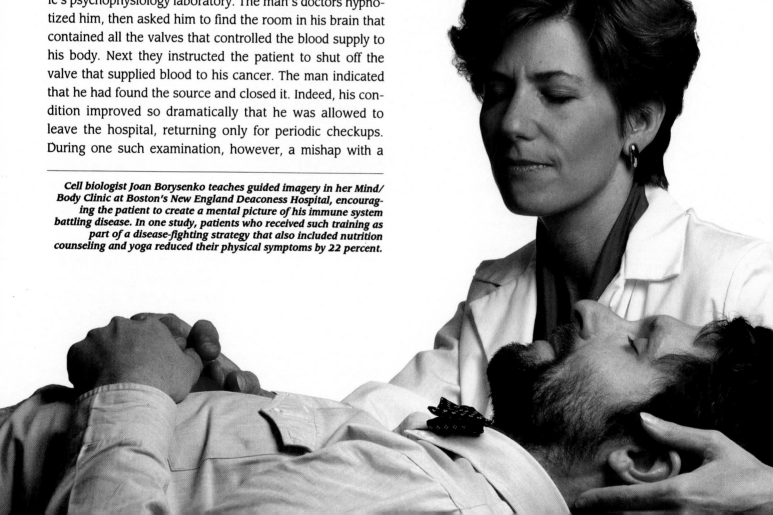

ganisms at a more rapid rate than when the test began. In Ohio, a healthy group of aged people given guided-imagery training boosted the count of their natural killer cells, while control groups without the training showed no increase. Imaging also has successfully been used to relieve chronic pain. Several specific images have been found particularly helpful for this purpose. One goes generically by the name "glove anesthesia." The patient is instructed to anesthetize one or both hands mentally, perhaps by imagining the hand being slipped into a very thick glove or by envisioning it being thrust into a bucket filled with a potent pain-killing solution. After the hand feels numb, the patient is told to transfer that feeling of numbness to the area of the body that is in pain.

Another helpful image for pain sufferers is that of the dimming light switch, or rheostat. The patient is instructed to imagine a switch with one wire leading to the brain and others leading to the painful area of the body. The wires leading to the pain glow and vibrate—a visual symbol of the pain itself. The patient is then told to turn the rheostat slowly and dim the glow of the wires—thereby dimming the very real feelings of pain.

Much remains to be learned about how visualization and other psychic healing techniques work and how effective they truly are in the fight against disease. The evidence already in, however, is persuasive enough that many physicians have already integrated some of these methods into the practice of medicine. At Boston's New England Deaconess Hospital, for example, patients suffering from illnesses ranging from allergies to AIDS are encouraged to join the hospital's Mind/Body Clinic. There, under the direction of Dr. Herbert Benson, a cardiologist who has pioneered in the field of relaxation techniques, participants receive training in such behavioral therapies as relaxation, visualization, yoga, nutrition counseling, and attitude changing—unconventional, but perhaps essential, ways of taking charge of their health and aiding in their own recovery.

To be sure, most respected mind-body researchers emphasize that these therapies are best used in conjunction with the practices of conventional medicine. As Dr. Benson puts it, "There is no mind-body [substitute] for penicillin or surgery or digitalis. You can't replace modern medicine; that's an absurdity."

Some nations already incorporate alternative therapies in their medical systems. The French espouse homeopathy, aroma therapy, and sojourns at restorative spas. West Germany's health care system offers hydrotherapy, herbal medicine, and mud baths, in addition to homeopathy. (To be included in the German system, "fringe" therapies must prove only that they are harmless—they do not have to show efficacy.)

This may seem startling to those who have believed unswervingly in the power of medical science to fine-tune the engine that is the human body and even replace worn-out parts. But consider some statistics cited by Dr. Kerr L. White, retired deputy director for health services at the Rockefeller Foundation: In his foreword to *Medicine & Culture*, a 1988 survey of health systems, Kerr contended that only about 15 percent of modern medical treatments are "supported by objective scientific evidence that they do more good than harm. On the other hand, between 40 and 60 percent of all therapeutic benefits can be attributed to caring and concern, or what most people call 'love.' "

There is no doubt that humans are extraordinarily complex and interdependent beings who need support from one another, both in groups and individually. Human beings can also learn to tap inner resources to help cope with, and sometimes conquer, illness. But perhaps the most successful approach to health is one that employs all the strategies that seem to be effective—an approach that includes a network of support, a partnership with a trusted physician, and strong individual will. As the honored physician and humanitarian Albert Schweitzer once observed, "The witch doctor succeeds for the same reason all the rest of us succeed. Each patient carries his own doctor inside him. We are at our best when we give the doctor who resides within each patient a chance to go to work."

ACKNOWLEDGMENTS

The editors wish to thank these individuals and institutions for their assistance in the preparation of this volume:

Dr. Robert Ader, University of Rochester Medical Center, Rochester, New York; Dr. William John Alloway, Bethesda, Maryland; David Andrews, Christian Science Center, Boston; Joanne Apple, American College of Orgonomy, Princeton, New Jersey; Camille Bartus, R.N., Alexandria, Virginia; Professor Hans Bender, Institut für Grenzgebiete der Psychologie und Psychohygiene, Freiburg, West Germany; Dr. Alfred Benjamin, Santa Monica, California; Harold Benjamin, Wellness Community, Santa Monica, California; Dr. Daniel Benor, London; Dr. Herbert Benson, New England Deaconess Hospital, Boston; Dr. Joan Borysenko, New England Deaconess Hospital, Boston; Ramus Branch, The Harry Edwards Healing Sanctuary, Shere, Surrey, England; Giulio Brunner, "Giornale dei Misteri," Florence, Italy; Willard Caldwell, Ph.D., Washington, D.C.; Dr. Barrie Cassileth, University of Pennsylvania Hospital, Philadelphia; Jan Chrissafis, Silver Spring, Maryland; Nicholas Clarke-Lowes, The Society for Psychical Research, London; E. E. Missy Cochrane, Bethesda, Maryland; Dr. Nicholas Cohen, University of Rochester Medical Center, Rochester, New York; Dr. Sanford Cohen, University of Miami Medical Center, Florida; Tom Creed, Ph.D., St. John's University, Collegeville, Minnesota; Diana DiPinto, The Delawarr Laboratories, Oxford, England; Janice Ellicot, London; Oskar Estebany,

Montreal; Dr. Steve Fahrion, The Menninger Foundation, Topeka, Kansas; Professor Elena Filibeck, I.S.M.E.O., Rome; Dr. William Fitzhugh, Department of Anthropology, Smithsonian Institution, Washington, D.C.; Pierre Franchomme, Laboratoire Pranarom, Belvèze du Razès, France; Jane Fryer, Washington, D.C.; Joy Gardner, Freedom, California; Paola Giovetti, Modena, Italy; Steve Gottshalk, Christian Science Center, Boston; Bernard Grad, Ph.D., Montreal; Dr. Elmer Green, The Menninger Foundation, Topeka, Kansas; Michael Harris, Medical Sciences Division, Smithsonian Institution, Washington, D.C.; John Hubacher, Venice, California; Wallace Janssen, United States Food and Drug Administration, Rockville, Maryland; Dr. Liang Jinsheng, Beijing International Acupuncture Training Center, Beijing; Tom Johnson, Christian Science Center, Boston; Leslie Kaslof, Woodmere, New York; Professor Dolores Krieger, Port Chester, New York; Albert W. Kuhfeld, Ph.D., The Bakken Library and Museum of Electricity in Life, Minneapolis; Professor Andreas Lommel, Munich; Peter Mandel, Bruchsal, West Germany; Anne Mattison, *New Realities Magazine,* Washington, D.C.; Nicole Maxwell, Institute for Botanical Exploration, Mississippi State University, State College; Ian Miller, C. W. Daniel Co. Ltd., Saffron Walden, Essex, England; Eleanor O'Keeffe, The Society for Psychical Research, London; Dr. Rita Otto, Munich; Dr. Charles E. Paterno, Rumson, New Jersey; Dr. Daniel Pénoël,

Étrechy, France; Professor Luciano Petech, I.S.M.E.O., Rome; Dr. Mark Plotkin, World Wildlife Fund, Washington, D.C.; Flo Porter, Wellness Community, Santa Monica, California; Albert-Claude Quemoun, Paris; Dr. Janet Quinn, Denver; John Ramsell, The Dr. E. Bach Centre, Wallingford, Oxfordshire, England; Katrina Raphaell, The Crystal Academy of Advanced Healing Arts, Taos; Dr. Hubert Rosomoff, University of Miami, Florida; Marilyn Schlitz, San Antonio; John Senior, The Bakken Library and Museum of Electricity in Life, Minneapolis; Dr. Bernard Siegel, New Haven, Connecticut; Dr. Peter Skaffe, Santa Barbara, California; Howard Sochurek, New York; Roy Stemman, London; Dennis Stillings, Archaeus Project, St. Paul, Minnesota; Dr. Rolf Streichardt, Institut für Grenzgebiete der Psychologie und Psychohygiene, Freiburg, West Germany; Fraser Swift, The Wellcome Museum of the History of Medicine, London; Robert Tisserand, The Tisserand Aromatherapy Institute, Hove, East Sussex, England; Alberto Villoldo, Palo Alto, California; John Walker, The Radionics Association, Deddington, Oxfordshire, England; John Walmsley, Epsom, Surrey, England; Suzanne White, United States Food and Drug Administration, Rockville, Maryland; Barbara Williams, Hahnemann University, Philadelphia; Mietek and Margaret Wirkus, Bethesda, Maryland; Wang Yan, Foreign Affairs Office, Beijing International Acupuncture Training Center, Beijing; Pat and Mike Young, Alexandria, Virginia.

PICTURE CREDITS

The sources for the illustrations in this book are shown below. Credits from left to right are separated by semicolons; credits from top to bottom are separated by dashes.

Cover: Art by Bryan Leister. 1, 3, and initial alphabet: Art by John Drummond. 7: Art by Michael Hill. 8: Staatliches Museum für Völkerkunde, Munich. 9: Werner Forman Archive, London—American Museum of Natural History, courtesy The Smithsonian Institution. 11: Peter Skafte. 12, 13: Eric Valli, Saint-Jorioz, France. 14: Peter T. Furst, courtesy New York State Museum. 15: Courtesy The Wheelwright Museum of the American Indian, Santa Fe, New Mexico. 16: Dirk Reinartz/Stern, Hamburg, West Germany. 18: Victor Englebert, from *Peoples of the Wild; Aborigines of the Amazon Rain Forest,* Time-Life Books International, Ltd., 1982. 19: Philip Bennett. 21: Eric Valli, Saint-Jorioz, France, copied by Larry Sherer from *The Honey Hunters of Nepal,* by Eric Valli and Diane Summers, Harry N. Abrams, New York, 1988. 22, 23: Timm Rautert/Visum Archiv, Hamburg, West Germany. 24-26: Carole Devillers. 28, 29: Stephanie Maze © 1988/ Woodfin Camp, Inc. 30: The Granger Collection, New York. 31: Edgar Cayce Foundation, Virginia Beach, Virginia. 34: Ray Branch, The Harry Edwards Healing Sanctuary, Surrey, England. 35: Background photo, The Aldus Archive, London—The Topham Picture Library, Edenbridge, Kent, England. 37: Guy Lyon Playfair/Mary Evans Picture Library, London. 39: © Nathan Benn 1980/Woodfin Camp, Inc. 40: Toby Molenaar, Paris. 41: © Nathan Benn 1982/Woodfin Camp, Inc. 42, 43: Bryan and Cherry Alexander, Dorset, England; Dimis Argyropoulos, Athens. 45: Art by Michael Hill. 46: Wellcome Museum of the History of Medicine, London. 47: Art by John Drummond. 48: Henry Wolf © 1984 *DISCOVER.* 49: Loh Wen Kai, courtesy The Chinese Medical Train-

ing Institution, Kuala Lumpur, Malaysia. 50: Acupuncture Research Institute, Beijing. 52, 53: Xinhua News Pictures, Beijing, except background photo, © Nik Wheeler. 55: Andrew McClenaghan/Science Photo Library, London—courtesy The Ohashi Institute, New York. 56: The Wellcome Institute Library, London. 59: IL HWA American Corporation. 60: Photo by Meg Landsman © 1983. 62: V. Shumkov/ UNESCO Courier. 64: Roland and Sabrina Michaud, Paris. 65: Wellcome Museum of the History of Medicine, London. 67: P. J. Griffiths/Magnum Photos. 68: Shostal/Superstock. 69: Douglas Wetzstein/World & I Photos. 70, 71: Larry Sherer. 72: Navin Kumar Gallery, New York. 73: Ted Thai/ *TIME* magazine, © Time Inc. 75: Courtesy Georgetown University Hospital, Washington, D.C. 76: Courtesy NASA. 77: Courtesy Lee Kudrow, California Medical Clinic for Headache, Encino (3)—courtesy Mallinckrodt Institute of Radiology, St. Louis, Missouri; Howard Sochurek. 78: Thelma Moss/SPL/Photo Researchers, Inc. 79: Georges Hadjo, Paris. 80, 81: Courtesy Elizabeth Tansley, Chichester, West Sussex, England, from *Radionics Interface with the Ether Fields,* by David Tansley, C. W. Daniel Co., Ltd., Saffron Walden, Essex, England, 1980, except bottom right, Delawarr Laboratories, Oxford, England. 83: Art by Michael Hill. 84, 85: S. Salgado, Jr./Magnum Photos. 86: Roger Viollet, Paris. 88: The Bettmann Archive—Larry Sherer, courtesy Medical Sciences Division, National Museum of American History, Smithsonian Institution; courtesy The Bakken Library and Museum of Electricity in Life, Minneapolis, Minnesota. 89: Courtesy The New York Public Library, Astor, Lenox and Tilden Foundations—Larry Sherer, courtesy Medical Sciences Division, National Museum of American History, Smithsonian Institution. 91: Archives Tallandier, Paris. 92: Daily Telegraph Colour Library, London. 94: Pho-

to by John Larsen, © 1972, *New Realities,* L.P. 96, 97: Bryce Bond/Parabond. 98: Lloyd Wolf. 100: Kari Berggrav, courtesy American College of Orgonomy—Kari Berggrav from *Wilhelm Reich vs. the U.S.A.,* by Jerome Greenfield, W. W. Norton & Co., Inc., New York, 1974. 101: Rapho/Photo Researchers, Inc. 102: Jean-Guy Thibodeau, courtesy Bernard Grad—Cristal Photo, Quebec, courtesy Oskar Estebany. 103: Courtesy Bernard Grad. 105: Paul Rodriquez/*The Orange County Register.* 106: © 1988 Paul Fusco/Magnum Photos. 108: John Walmsley, Epsom, from *Awareness through Colour,* by Howard and Dorothy Sun, Prism Press, Bridport, Dorset, England, forthcoming. 109: Andrew Eccles/Rebus Inc. 110, 111: From *Crystal Healing,* by Katrina Raphaell, Aurora Press, Santa Fe, New Mexico, 1987—all stones courtesy of Mazi Artmine, subsidiary of the Twillman Co., except for carnelian, bicolored watermelon tourmaline, azurite, and bloodstone, courtesy Olde Towne Gemstones, all photographed by Larry Sherer. 113: Paul Biddle and Tim Malyon/Science Photo Library, London. 114: Larry Sherer. 117: Art by Michael Hill. 118: Steve Shapiro/Sygma. 120: Courtesy the Archives, Hahnemann University, Philadelphia, Pennsylvania. 121: Courtesy the Archives, Hahnemann University, Philadelphia, Pennsylvania; Henry Groskinsky from *Library of Health; Prudent Use of Medicines,* Time-Life Books, Inc., 1981. 122: Roger Viollet, Paris. 123: The Hulton Picture Library, London. 125: The Granger Collection, New York. 127: Michael Abramson/ Onyx. 128, 129: Anne Jill Leonard/*Halo* magazine. 130, 131: Gail Mooney and Tom Kelly/© 1982, *DISCOVER.* 132, 133: Paul Fusco/Magnum Photos. 134: Courtesy Louise Hay House, Inc., Santa Monica, California. 136: Courtesy The Menninger Foundation, Topeka, Kansas. 137: Nicholas Blair, courtesy Herbert Benson. 138: Brownie Harris.

BIBLIOGRAPHY

Ader, Robert, and Nicholas Cohen, "Behaviorally Conditioned Immunosuppression." *Psychosomatic Medicine,* July-August 1975.

Aikman, Lonnelle, *Nature's Healing Arts: From Folk Medicine to Modern Drugs.* Washington, D.C.: National Geographic Society, 1977.

"Ambrose & Olga Worrall in Interview: Two of the World's Most Respected Healers." *Psychic,* April 1972.

Bach, Edward, M.D., and F. J. Wheeler, M.D., *The Bach Flower Remedies.* New Canaan, Conn.: Keats, 1979.

Barrett, Stephen, "Homeopathy: Is It Medicine?" *Skeptical Inquirer,* fall 1987.

Barrett, Stephen, and Gilda Knight, eds., *The Health Robbers: How to Protect Your Money and Your Life.* Philadelphia: George F. Stickley, 1976.

Bartlett, Laile E., *PSI Trek.* New York: McGraw-Hill, 1981.

Bishop, George, *Faith Healing: God or Fraud?* Los Angeles: Sherbourne Press, 1967.

Bloom, William L., Jr., John L. Hollenbach, and James A. Morgan, eds., *Medical Radiographic Technic.* Springfield, Ill.: Charles C. Thomas, 1972.

Borysenko, Joan, with Larry Rothstein, *Minding the Body, Mending the Mind.* Reading, Mass.: Addison-Wesley, 1987.

Bramly, Serge, *The Teachings of Maria-Jose, Mother of the Gods.* Transl. by Meg Bogin. New York: St. Martin's Press, 1977.

Branch, Ramus, *Harry Edwards.* Shere, Surrey, England: Burrows Lea, 1982.

Brennan, Barbara Ann, *Hands of Light: A Guide to Healing through the Human Energy Field.* New York: Bantam Books, 1987.

Brody, Jane E.:
Jane Brody's The New York Times Guide to Personal Health. New York: Times Books, 1982.
"Laying On of Hands Gains New Respect." *The New York Times,* March 26, 1985.

Cavendish, Richard, ed., *Man, Myth & Magic.* New York: Marshall Cavendish, 1983.

Cerutti, Edwina, *Olga Worrall: Mystic with the Healing Hands.* New York: Harper & Row, 1975.

Chancellor, Philip M., ed. and comp., *Illustrated Handbook of the Bach Flower Remedies.* Saffron Walden, Essex, England: C. W. Daniel, 1971.

Clark, Philip E., and Mary Jo Clark, "Therapeutic Touch: Is There a Scientific Basis for the Practice?" In *Examining Holistic Medicine,* ed. by Douglas Stalker and Clark Glymour. Buffalo, N.Y.: Prometheus Books, 1985.

Cohen, Sherry Suib, *The Magic of Touch.* New York: Harper & Row, 1987.

Cousins, Norman, *Anatomy of an Illness As Perceived by the Patient.* New York: W. W. Norton, 1979.

Cunningham, Alastair J., "Mind, Body, and Immune Response." In *Psychoneuroimmunology,* ed. by Robert Ader. New York: Academic Press, 1981.

Davis, Andrew Jackson, *The Harbinger of Health.* Boston: Banner of Light Publishing Co., 1879.

Day, Langston, and George de la Warr, *New Worlds beyond the Atom.* New York: Devin-Adair, 1963.

De Courcy, Anne, "Are You a Hypnotic Subject?" *Telegraph Sunday Magazine* (London), March 3, 1985.

Devillers, Carole, "Haiti's Voodoo Pilgrimages of Spirits and Saints." *National Geographic,* March 1985.

Dubrick, Michael A., "Historical Perspectives on the Use of Herbal Preparations to Promote Health." *Journal of Nutrition,* July 1986.

Eastman, Yvette, *Touchpoint: Reflexology, the First Steps.*
Campbell River, B.C., Canada: Ptarmigan Press, 1985.

"East Meets West to Balance Immunologic Yin and Yang." *Journal of the American Medical Association,* January 27, 1984.

Eden, Jerome, *Animal Magnetism and the Life Energy.* Hicksville, N.Y.: Exposition Press, 1974.

Eisenberg, David, M.D., and Thomas Lee Wright, *Encounters with Qi.* New York: W. W. Norton, 1985.

Fenton, William N., *The False Faces of the Iroquois.* Norman, Okla.: University of Oklahoma Press, 1987.

Fitzhugh, William W., and Aron Crowell, *Crossroads of Continents.* Washington, D.C.: Smithsonian Institution, 1988.

Flammonde, Paris, *The Mystic Healers.* New York: Stein and Day, 1974.

Frank, Jerome D., M.D., *Persuasion and Healing.* Baltimore: Johns Hopkins Press, 1973.

Friedman, Milton, "From Poland with Prana." *New Realities,* July-August 1987.

Fuller, Robert C., *Mesmerism and the American Cure of Souls.* Philadelphia: University of Pennsylvania Press, 1982.

Gaines, Judith, "Romancing the Stones: A Look into the Crystal Craze." *Boston Globe Magazine,* April 24, 1988.

Gallagher, Winifred, "The Healing Touch." *American Health,* October 1988.

Garber, Janet Serlin, *Rasputin: The Mysterious Monk.* New York: Contemporary Perspectives, 1979.

Gardner, Frank H., and Louis K. Diamond, "Autoerythrocyte Sensitization." *Journal of Hematology,* July 1955.

Gardner, Joy, *Color and Crystals: A Journey through the Chakras.* Freedom, Calif.: Crossing Press, 1988.

Gardner, Martin:
The New Age: Notes of a Fringe Watcher. Buffalo, N.Y.: Prometheus Books, 1988.
"Reich the Rainmaker: The Orgone Obsession." *Skeptical Inquirer,* fall 1988.

Gavzer, Bernard, "Why Do Some People Survive AIDS?" *Parade Magazine,* September 18, 1988.

Geis, Larry, and Alta Picchi Kelly, *The New Healers: Healing the Whole Person.* Berkeley, Calif.: New Dimensions, 1980.

Gelman, David, and Mary Hager, "Body and Soul." *Newsweek,* November 7, 1988.

Gerber, Richard, M.D., *Vibrational Medicine: New Choices for Healing Ourselves.* Santa Fe: Bear & Co., 1988.

Gillespie, Marcia, "Healer Meyerson." *Ms.,* December 1985.

Gimbel, Theo:
Form, Sound, Colour and Healing. Saffron Walden, Essex, England: C. W. Daniel, 1987.
Healing through Colour. Saffron Walden, Essex, England: C. W. Daniel, 1980.

Goldstein, Laura, "Feeling Guru-vy." *Dossier,* September 1987.

Grad, Bernard R.:
"Orgonotic Functions in Healing by Touch." *Journal of Orgonomy,* Vol. 20, Issue 2, 1986.
"Some Biological Effects of the 'Laying On of Hands': A Review of Experiments with Animals and Plants." *The Journal of the American Society for Psychical Research,* April 1965.

Grady, Denise, "AIDS Survivors: Beating the Odds." *American Health,* September 1988.

Green, Elmer, and Alyce Green, *Beyond Biofeedback.* New York: Melroyd Lawrence, 1977.
Hafen, Brent Q., and Kathryn J. Frandsen, *From Acupuncture to Yoga: Alternative Methods of Healing.* Englewood Cliffs, N.J.: Prentice-Hall, 1983.

Hand, Wayland D., ed., *American Folk Medicine: A Symposium.* Berkeley, Calif.: University of California Press, 1976.

Hartmann, Franz, M.D., *The Life of Paracelsus.* San Diego: Wizards Bookshelf, 1985.

Hathaway, Bruce, "Circuity, Wizards, and New Agers Alike Can Get Good Vibes from Quartz." *Smithsonian,* November 1988.

Hay, Louise L., *Heal Your Body.* Santa Monica: Hay House, 1988.

Hildegard of Bingen and Matthew Fox, *Illuminations of Hildegard of Bingen.* Santa Fe: Bear & Co., 1985.

Hines, Terence, *Pseudoscience and the Paranormal.* Buffalo, N.Y.: Prometheus Books, 1988.

Hunt, Roland, *The Seven Keys to Color Healing.* San Francisco: Harper & Row, 1971.

Hutton, J. Bernard, *Healing Hands.* London: W. H. Allen, 1978.

Inglis, Brian, and Ruth West, *The Alternative Health Guide.* New York: Alfred A. Knopf, 1983.

Ishida, Yasuo, "Acupuncture Today." *Southern Medical Journal,* July 1988.

Iyengar, B. K. S., *Light on Yoga.* New York: Schocken Books, 1976.

Jaggi, O. P., *Yogic and Tantric Medicine.* New Delhi: Atma Ram, 1973.

Jarvis, D. C., *Folk Medicine: A Vermont Doctor's Guide to Good Health.* Don Mills, Ontario, Canada: George J. McCloud, 1978.

Johnson, Dirk, "Therapists Offer Relief by Putting Patient on the Right Scent." *The New York Times,* November 8, 1988.

Kaptchuk, Ted J., *The Web That Has No Weaver.* New York: Congdon & Weed, 1983.

Karp, Reba Ann, *Edgar Cayce Encyclopedia of Healing.* New York: Warner Books, 1986.

Katz, Naomi, "For Love of a Sea." *Américas,* July-August 1986.

Keville, Kathi, "Aromatherapy: Healing the Mind and Body with Essential Oils." *Vegetarian Times,* November 1988.

King, Francis, "To Hell and Back." *The Unexplained* (London), Vol. 12, Issue 138.

Kingston, Jeremy, *Healing without Medicine.* Garden City, N.Y.: Doubleday, 1976.

Knight, Nancy, *Pain and Its Relief* (exhibition catalog). Washington, D.C.: Smithsonian Institution, 1983.

Korn, Errol R., and Karen Johnson, *Visualization.* Homewood, Ill.: Dow Jones-Irwin, 1983.

Krieger, Dolores:
Living the Therapeutic Touch. New York: Dodd, Mead, 1987.
The Therapeutic Touch: How to Use Your Hands to Help or to Heal. New York: Prentice Hall, 1979.

Krier, Beth Ann, "An Evening with Louise Hay." *Los Angeles Times,* March 2, 1988.

Krippner, Stanley, and Alberto Villoldo, *The Realms of Healing.* Millbrae, Calif.: Celestial Arts, 1976.

Krippner, Stanley, and Daniel Rubin, eds., *The Kirlian Aura.* Garden City, N.Y.: Doubleday, 1974.

Kubie, Lawrence S., "The Problem of Specificity in the Psychosomatic Process." In *The Psychosomatic Concept in Psychoanalysis,* ed. by Felix Deutsch, M.D. New York: International Universities Press, 1953.

Kurtz, Howard, "Cracking Drug Addiction." *The Washington Post, September 5, 1988.

Kushi, Michio, and Aveline Kushi, *Macrobiotic Diet*. Ed. by Alex Jack. Toyko: Japan Publications, 1985.

"Laboratory Tests Show Patients Receive 'Energy' from Healer." *Psychic News* (London), January 19, 1974.

Langguth, A. J., *Macumba: White and Black Magic in Brazil*. New York: Harper & Row, 1975.

Langone, John, "Acupuncture: New Respect for an Ancient Remedy." *Discover*, August 1984.

Levy, Sandra M., et al., "Survival Hazards Analysis in First Recurrent Breast Cancer Patients: Seven-Year Follow-Up." *Psychosomatic Medicine*, April 1988.

Lewis, Angelo John, "The Art of Aromatherapy: Healing with Essential Oils." *East West*, October 1988.

Lidell, Lucy, with Narayani Rabinovitch and Giris Rabinovitch, *The Sivananda Companion to Yoga*. New York: Simon & Schuster, 1983.

Linder, Lawrence, "The New, Improved Macrobiotic Diet." *American Health*, May 1988.

Locke, Steven, M.D., and Douglas Colligan, *The Healer Within*. New York: New American Library, 1986.

Lommel, Andreas, *Shamanism: The Beginnings of Art*. Transl. by Michael Bullock. New York: McGraw-Hill, 1967.

Lowen, Alexander, M.D., *Bioenergetics*. New York: Penguin Books, 1975.

Luthe, Wolfgang, "Autogenic Training: Method, Research and Application in Medicine." In *Biofeedback and Self-Control*, ed. by Joe Kamiya. Chicago: Aldine-Atherton, 1971.

Lyons, Albert S., M.D., and R. Joseph Petrucelli, M.D., *Medicine: An Illustrated History*. New York: Harry N. Abrams, 1978.

McKenna, Dennis J., and Terence K. McKenna, *The Invisible Landscape*. New York: Seabury Press, 1975.

Maharishi Ayur-Veda™ Medical Center, *Patient Education Program* (general information packet). Washington, D.C.: Maharishi Ayurveda Corporation of America, 1987.

Maier, H. John, Jr., "Brazil's Black Magic." *Travel Holiday*, March 1987.

Mann, W. Edward, *Orgone, Reich and Eros: Wilhelm Reich's Theory of Life Energy*. New York: Simon & Schuster, 1973.

Marais, Gill, "Ayurveda: India's Life Science." *The World and I*, February 1988.

Marchenay, Philippe, *L'Homme et l'Abeille*. Paris: Berger-Levrault, 1979.

Moore, Michael C., and Lynda J. Moore, *The Complete Handbook of Holistic Health*. Englewood Cliffs, N.J.: Prentice-Hall, 1983.

Morrell, Virginia, "Jungle Rx." *International Wildlife*, May-June 1988.

Moss, Thelma, *The Body Electric*. Los Angeles: J. P. Tarcher, 1979.

Murdock, Barbara Scott, *The Bakken: A Library and Museum of Electricity in Life* (exhibition catalog). Minneapolis: The Bakken, 1986.

Murthy, N. Anjneya, and D. P. Pandy, *Ayurvedic Cure for Common Diseases*. Delhi: Orient Paperbacks, 1982.

Needham, Joseph, *Science in Traditional China*. Cambridge, Mass.: Harvard University Press, 1981.

Newman, Barbara, *Sister of Wisdom: St. Hildegard's Theology of the Feminine*. Berkeley, Calif.: University of California Press, 1987.

Nicholson, Shirley, comp., *Shamanism: An Expanded View of Reality*. Wheaton, Ill.: Theosophical Publishing House, 1987.

Nolen, William A., *Healing: A Doctor in Search of a Miracle*. New York: Random House, 1974.

Ohashi, Wataru, *Do-It-Yourself Shiatsu*. Ed. by Vicki Lindner. New York: E. P. Dutton, 1976.

Orne, Martin T., and David F. Dinges, "Hypnosis." In *Textbook of Pain*, ed. by Patrick D. Wall and Ronald Melzack. Edinburgh, Scotland: Churchill Livingstone, 1984.

Ornstein, Robert, and David Sobel:
"Can You Psych Yourself into Good Health?" *Glamour*, August 1987. *The Healing Brain*. New York: Simon & Schuster, 1987.

Ornstein, Robert, and Richard F. Thompson, *The Amazing Brain*. Boston: Houghton Mifflin, 1984.

Page, Jake, "Are Crystals Stones of Enlightenment and Healing or Just a Bunch of Pretty Rocks?" *Omni*, October 1987.

Payer, Lynn, *Medicine & Culture*. New York: Henry Holt, 1988.

Pelletier, Kenneth R., *Mind as Healer, Mind as Slayer*. New York: Merloyd Lawrence, 1977.

Podmore, Frank, *From Mesmer to Christian Science*. New Hyde Park, N.Y.: University Books, 1963.

Portugal, Franklin H., "Medical Imaging: The Technology of Body Art." *High Technology*, November-December 1982.

Quinn, Janet, "Therapeutic Touch." *New Realities*, May-June 1987.

Randi, James:
The Faith Healers. Buffalo, N.Y.: Prometheus Books, 1983.
Flim-Flam!: Psychics, ESP, Unicorns and Other Delusions. Buffalo, N.Y.: Prometheus Books, 1987.

Raphaell, Katrina:
Crystal Enlightenment. Santa Fe: Aurora Press, 1985.
Crystal Healing. Santa Fe: Aurora Press, 1987.

Reid, Daniel P., *Chinese Herbal Medicine*. Boston: Shambhala, 1987.

Reuben, Carolyn, "Healing Your Life with Louise Hay." *East West*, June 1988.

Rinzler, Carol Ann, *The Dictionary of Medical Folklore*. New York: Thomas Y. Crowell, 1979.

Rodman, Selden, "African Brazil and Its Cults." *Américas*, June 1975.

Rogers, Spencer, *The Shaman, His Symbols and Healing Magic*. Springfield, Ill.: Charles C. Thomas, 1982.

Rose, Louis, *Faith Healing*. Ed. by Bryan Morgan. New York: Penguin Books, 1971.

Roth, Nancy:
"Duchenne and the Accuracy Esthetic." *Medical Instrumentation*, September-October 1979.
"Electroresuscitation and the Occult." *Medical Instrumentation*, March-April 1980.

Schaefer, Gerschen L., M.D., Sharon Boothby, and Nancy Marchand, "Is There a Place for Kirlian Photography in the Practice of Medicine." Scientific Exhibit, California Medical Association's 111th Annual Session (Anaheim, Calif.), March 1982.

Schiegl, Heinz, *Healing Magnetism: The Transference of Vital Force*. York Beach, Maine: Samuel Weiser, 1983.

Schleifer, Steven J., et al., "Suppression of Lymphocyte Stimulation Following Bereavement." *Journal of the American Medical Association*, July 15, 1983.

Schmale, A. H., and H. Iker, "Hopelessness as a Predictor of Cervical Cancer." *Society of Science & Medicine* (Great Britain), Vol. 5, 1971.

Seamens, Dan, comp., "Healing with Honeybees." *East West*, October 1988.

Shepard, Leslie A., ed., *Encyclopedia of Occultism & Para-psychology*. 3 vols. Detroit: Gale Research, 1985.

Siegel, Bernie S., M.D., *Love, Medicine & Miracles*. New York: Harper & Row, 1986.

Skafte, Peter, "Following the Woman-Faced Deer: The Inner World of Nepalese Shamanism." *Shaman's Drum*, summer 1988.

Skrabanek, Petr, "Acupuncture: Past, Present, and Future." In *Examining Holistic Medicine*, ed. by Douglas Stalker and Clark Glymour. Buffalo, N.Y.: Prometheus Books, 1985.

Smilgis, Martha, "Rock Power for Health and Wealth." *Time*, January 19, 1987.

Sochurek, Howard, "Medicine's New Vision." *National Geographic*, January 1987.

Squires, Sally, "Visions to Boost Immunity." *American Health*, July-August 1987.

Stalker, Douglas, and Clark Glymour, eds., *Examining Holistic Medicine*. Buffalo, N.Y.: Prometheus Books, 1985.

Stearn, Jess, *Edgar Cayce: The Sleeping Prophet*. New York: Doubleday, 1967.

Steiner, Lee R., *Psychic Self-Healing for Psychological Problems*. Englewood Cliffs, N.J.: Prentice-Hall, 1977.

Strehlow, Wighard, and Gottfried Hertzka, M.D., *Hildegard of Bingen's Medicine*. Transl. by Karin Strehlow. Santa Fe: Bear & Co., 1988.

Sugrue, Thomas, *There Is a River: The Story of Edgar Cayce*. New York: Dell, 1970.

Susac, Andrew, *Paracelsus: Monarch of Medicine*. Garden City, N.Y.: Doubleday, 1969.

Takahashi, Masaru, and Stephen Brown, *Qigong for Health*. Toyko: Japan Publications, 1986.

Tansley, David V., *Radionics: Interface with the Ether-Fields*. Saffron Walden, Essex, England: C. W. Daniel, 1975.

Tansley, David V., with Malcolm Rae and Aubrey T. Westlake, *Dimensions of Radionics*. Saffron Walden, Essex, England: C. W. Daniel, 1977.

Taylor, John, *Science and the Supernatural*. New York: E. P. Dutton, 1980.

Thakkur, Chandrashekhar, *Introduction to Ayurveda (Basic Indian Medicine)*. Bombay: Ancient Wisdom Publication, 1965.

Tisserand, Robert B., *The Art of Aromatherapy*. Rochester, Vt.: Destiny Books, 1977.

U.S. Department of Health and Human Services, *Biofeedback* (National Institute of Mental Health Plain Talk series). Ed. by Ruth Kay. ADM 83-1273. Rockville, Md.: Alcohol, Drug Abuse, and Mental Health Administration, 1983.

Veith, Ilza, *Huang Ti Nei Ching Su Wen*. Baltimore: Williams and Wilkins, 1949.

Watkins, Arleen J., and William S. Bickel, "A Study of the Kirlian Effect." *Skeptical Inquirer*, spring 1986.

Weil, Andrew, *Health and Healing*. Boston: Houghton Mifflin, 1983.

Wilson, Colin, *Mysterious Powers*. London: Aldus Books, 1975.

Wingerson, Lois, "Training the Mind to Heal." *Discover*, May 1982.

Wolman, Benjamin B., ed., *Handbook of Parapsychology*. Jefferson, N.C.: McFarland, 1977.

Wynder, Ernst L., M.D., ed., *The Book of Health*. New York: Franklin Watts, 1981.

Yamamoto, Shizuko, *Barefoot Shiatsu*. Toyko: Japan Publications, 1979.

Young, James Harvey, *The Medical Messiahs: A Social History of Health Quackery in Twentieth-Century America*. Princeton, N.J.: Princeton University Press, 1967.

INDEX

Time-Life Books Inc.
is a wholly owned subsidiary of
TIME INCORPORATED

Editor-in-Chief: Jason McManus
Chairman and Chief Executive Officer: J. Richard Munro
President and Chief Operating Officer: N. J. Nicholas, Jr.
Editorial Director: Richard B. Stolley

THE TIME INC. BOOK COMPANY
President and Chief Executive Officer: Kelso F. Sutton
President, Time Inc. Books Direct: Christopher T. Linen

TIME-LIFE BOOKS INC.

EDITOR: George Constable
Executive Editor: Ellen Phillips
Director of Design: Louis Klein
Director of Editorial Resources: Phyllis K. Wise
Editorial Board: Russell B. Adams, Jr., Dale M. Brown,
Roberta Conlan, Thomas H. Flaherty, Lee Hassig,
Donia Ann Steele, Rosalind Stubenberg
Director of Photography and Research:
John Conrad Weiser
Assistant Director of Editorial Resources: Elise Ritter Gibson

PRESIDENT: John M. Fahey, Jr.
Senior Vice Presidents: Robert M. DeSena, James L. Mercer,
Paul R. Stewart, Joseph J. Ward
Vice Presidents: Stephen L. Bair, Stephen L. Goldstein,
Juanita T. James, Andrew P. Kaplan, Carol Kaplan,
Susan J. Maruyama, Robert H. Smith
Supervisor of Quality Control: James King

PUBLISHER: Joseph J. Ward

Editorial Operations
Copy Chief: Diane Ullius
Production: Celia Beattie
Library: Louise D. Forstall

Library of Congress Cataloging in Publication Data
Powers of Healing / the editors of Time-Life Books.
    p. cm.—(Mysteries of the unknown)
Bibliography: p.
Includes index.
ISBN 0-8094-6356-3. ISBN 0-8094-6357-1 (lib. bdg.)
1. Healing. 2. Mental healing. 3. Mind and body.
I. Time-Life Books. II. Series.
RZ401.P89 1989
615.8'5—dc19   89-4415 CIP

The information in this book cannot and should not
replace the advice of a doctor. In the event of illness, you
should consult a qualified health professional.

MYSTERIES OF THE UNKNOWN

SERIES DIRECTOR: Russell B. Adams, Jr.
Series Administrator: Myrna Traylor-Herndon
Designer: Herbert H. Quarmby

Editorial Staff for *Powers of Healing*
Associate Editors: Sara Schneidman (pictures);
Janet Cave (text)
Text Editors: Laura Foreman, Jim Hicks
Researchers: Constance Contreras, Sarah D. Ince,
Elizabeth Ward
Staff Writer: Marfé Ferguson Delano
Assistant Designer: Susan M. Gibas
Copy Coordinators: Mary Beth Oelkers-Keegan,
Jarelle S. Stein
Picture Coordinator: Ruth J. Moss
Editorial Assistant: Donna Fountain

Special Contributors: Christine Hinze (London, picture
research); Paul R. Edholm (lead research); Ruth J. Moss,
Janis K. Oppelt, Patricia A. Paterno, Evelyn Prettyman
(research); George Daniels, Lydia Preston Hicks, Robert
Kiener, Gregory McGruder, Wendy Murphy, Susan Perry,
Nancy Shuker, Daniel Stashower, Erwin Washington,
F. Peter Wigginton (text); John Drummond (design); Hazel
Blumberg-McKee (index)

Correspondents: Elisabeth Kraemer-Singh (Bonn), Vanessa
Kramer (London), Christina Lieberman (New York); Maria
Vincenza Aloisi (Paris), Ann Natanson (Rome)
Valuable assistance was also provided by Mirka Gondicas
(Athens); Angelika Lemmer (Bonn); Judy Aspinall
(London); Simmi Dhanda, Deepak Puri (New Delhi);
Elizabèth Brown, Cindy Joyce (New York); Ann Wise
(Rome); Lawrence Chang (Taipei); Dick Berry, Mieko
Ikeda (Tokyo).

The Consultants:
Marcello Truzzi, the general consultant for the series, is a
professor of sociology at Eastern Michigan University. He
is also director of the Center for Scientific Anomalies
Research (CSAR) and editor of its journal, the *Zetetic
Scholar.* Dr. Truzzi, who considers himself a "constructive
skeptic" with regard to claims of the paranormal, works
through the CSAR to produce dialogues between critics
and proponents of unusual scientific claims.

John Allee is an acupuncturist and qigong instructor at the
Taoist Health Institute in Washington, D.C. He holds a
Ph.D. from Medicina Alternativa, an international teaching
and research institution established in 1962 by the World
Health Organization, and is currently writing a book on
Taoist longevity techniques.

Joan Halifax, an authority on shamanic traditions, is an
author, teacher, and medical anthropologist. She served
on the faculties of Columbia University, University of Miami School of Medicine, and Harvard University. She has
written a number of books on shamanism, including *Shamanic Voices* and *Shaman, the Wounded Healer,* and as-
sisted mythologist Joseph Campbell on his *Way of the Animal Powers.*

Nancy Kime Lonsdorf, M.D., practices Ayurvedic medicine
at the Maharishi Ayur-Veda Medical Center in Washington, D.C. She received her medical degree from Johns
Hopkins University School of Medicine and completed her
residence training at Stanford University School of Medicine. She has studied Ayurvedic health care extensively in
India and the U.S. and has lectured widely on the subject.

Other Publications:

AMERICAN COUNTRY
VOYAGE THROUGH THE UNIVERSE
THE THIRD REICH
THE TIME-LIFE GARDENER'S GUIDE
TIME FRAME
FIX IT YOURSELF
FITNESS, HEALTH & NUTRITION
SUCCESSFUL PARENTING
HEALTHY HOME COOKING
UNDERSTANDING COMPUTERS
LIBRARY OF NATIONS
THE ENCHANTED WORLD
THE KODAK LIBRARY OF CREATIVE PHOTOGRAPHY
GREAT MEALS IN MINUTES
THE CIVIL WAR
PLANET EARTH
COLLECTOR'S LIBRARY OF THE CIVIL WAR
THE EPIC OF FLIGHT
THE GOOD COOK
WORLD WAR II
HOME REPAIR AND IMPROVEMENT
THE OLD WEST

TIME LIFE ®

*For information on and a full description of any of the Time-
Life Books series listed above, please call 1-800-621-7026 or
write:*
Reader Information
Time-Life Customer Service
P.O. Box C-32068
Richmond, Virginia 23261-2068

This volume is one of a series that examines the history
and nature of seemingly paranormal phenomena. Other
books in the series include:

Time-Life Books Inc. offers a wide range of fine record-
ings, including a *Rock 'n' Roll Era* series. For subscription
information, call 1-800-621-7026 or write Time-Life
Music, P.O. Box C-32068, Richmond, Virginia 23261-2068.